the BAD BACK MANUAL

Intelligent 24 Hour Solutions to Correct
Posture & Heal Back Pain

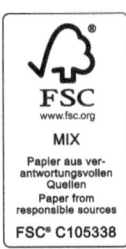

Bibliografische Information der Deutschen Nationalbibliothek:

Die Deutsche Nationalbibliothek verzeichnet diese Publikation in der
Deutschen Nationalbibliografie; detaillierte bibliografische Daten sind im
Internet über http://dnb.dnb.de abrufbar.

Herstellung und Verlag: BoD – Books on Demand, Norderstedt

ISBN: 9783837081558

DISCLAIMER

This book was written with the intention of providing you with a different, very personal, point of view on health issues, in particular back pain and other posture related musculoskeletal pains.

This book is not a substitute for a doctor or GP and you should not go against the recommendations of your health practitioner.

The author and the editor decline all responsibility for any adverse effects resulting directly or indirectly from advice, opinions or exercises contained in this book.

CONTENTS

HOW TO READ THIS BOOK

This book was written straight from the heart and is quite blunt. Please remember that any criticism is not aimed at you personally, dear reader. When I state that an exercise or habit is detrimental to posture and causes back pain, that does not mean that the person doing it is intellectually challenged.

You can only be an expert at so many things in life and it may just so happen that anatomy, biomechanics, ergonomics and posture are not on everyone's list.

This is true even if you are a health professional. I know many wonderful and competent doctors and therapists who do a great job every day. Many of the things I describe here are simply not on the curriculum of most medical schools.

So don't beat yourself up if you have been doing it wrong all those years!

In order to keep this book user-friendly and easy to read, I have avoided using footnotes and quoting from studies. When it comes to simple things like posture and back pain, I believe in the importance of logical arguments, not the authority of individual studies.

Sometimes, in order to make a point, I recommend "exercises". These exercises shouldn't be part of a daily routine, like running or weight lifting. They are designed to help you understand an argument that is being made.

In my experience, this *physical understanding* from experience is often more convincing and useful than purely logical reasoning.

I therefore suggest you do these exercises even if you have fully understood the point that is being made.

Don't hesitate to check out my youtube channel[1], where you will find demonstrations of exercises for better sitting and walking. I will directly refer you to some of my videos at certain points in the book.

I am also the author of a video course called "Improve Your Posture and Get Rid of Your Back Pain!" with more than 40 exercises to improve posture and alleviate back pain.

The course has helped hundreds of students improve their posture and alleviate their back pain and has received outstanding ratings and satisfaction levels. You can find out more about it at the end of the book (and get a discount).

TLDR

Each chapter is summed up with a TLDR (too long, didn't read), which summarizes the key points that have been made. This can be helpful whether you are looking for a specific piece of information or just revising the content of a chapter.

---

[1] https://www.youtube.com/user/senmoticfrance

PREFACE

Pain is youth leaving the body.
Unattributed

Think not only about curing back pain; think also about how to stop causing it. Obvious causes for back pain you must address first.

1 STEP FORWARD – 23 STEPS BACK?

An old joke tells the story of Dave, who prays to God every night asking to win the lottery. Dave prays to win the lottery every snight for twenty years – without success. Undeterred, he continues to pray, "God, please let me win the lottery!" One evening his prayer is interrupted by a heavenly voice: "GIVE YOURSELF A CHANCE AND BUY A TICKET, MATE!"

From the point of view of a therapist, most people go about fighting back pain the way Dave goes about winning the lottery: They fail to do the most important thing to resolve back pain, i.e. to stop causing it in the first place. Instead they spend an incredible amount of (mostly wasted) energy trying to deal with the consequences.

Some people use painkillers, others do yoga, stretching exercises, strength training, massage and so on. But this is as effective as trying to find good food supplements to support weight loss instead of just cutting out the burgers and fries.

This book is about the changes you must make, the habits you must kick, to get rid of your back pain. *Must* is a strong word, but throughout the book you will see how pointless doing posture correction exercises is, if your chair or your shoes keep killing your back all day long.

Knowing about these things is, of course, not enough on its own. This book can only help you if you implement these changes.

SIMPLE QUESTIONS

Sometimes simple questions are the most difficult to answer. Why, for example, do so many people experience back pain? It is not, after all, a virus that spreads like the flu or a bacteria that we are exposed to through food poisoning. Is there a basic weakness in the design of human beings that makes back pain inevitable?

Another simple question is: Why does back pain not heal spontaneously and then never come back? After all, we can cut our skin or break a bone and then the body heals itself, often within hours or days, but in weeks at the most.

Why do humans encounter back problems often, even within the first third of their lives, whilst other species do not?

What is even more confusing about back pain is the sheer number of possible remedies - even in traditional medicine. Some doctors recommend physical therapy, some just sports. Others will actually freeze the nerve endings in your lower back or inject painkillers with a needle, and that's before they even start talking about operations.

This variety of treatments is particularly confusing when you consider that with the flu or a fever, doctor's recommendations are pretty much the same all over the globe.

If you are reading this book, the chances are that you are like eighty percent of the population in that you experience back pain at least occasionally. Chances are also, that whatever cure you have tried in the past, your back pain comes back at least once a year. It is even quite likely that you experience it once a month.

"Pain is youth leaving the body" - and back pain, in particular, is so dangerous because it is often the beginning of a vicious circle. In order to avoid pain or injury, patients gradually stop doing activities like sports or spontaneous movements like jumping over a fence. After a few years, they actually become stiffer and incapable of those movements. "Use it or lose it" – everybody knows this to be true. Things that everybody knows to be true are usually wrong, but this is an exception to prove the rule. Trust me on this one.

Fighting back pain, therefore, is not just about avoiding pain. It is also about maintaining the multitude and amplitude of your movements. A person who can still move spontaneously and without fear of getting hurt isn't old – no matter his or her age.

Back to our initial question: Are humans doomed by design to experience back pain? No, a healthy, normal spine is not poorly designed. Of course, some people are born with scoliosis or other problems that will invariably lead to back pain. But these unlucky few only represent a small minority of bad back cases. Most back problems are lifestyle problems that can be treated.

In fact, the variety of treatments suggests that the causes of back pain are either not entirely understood, or else they are very difficult to identify in each patient.

I will argue that both assumptions are true. Pain is, as they say, mostly in our heads, and sometimes doctors and therapists are at a complete loss to put a finger on the reason why a seemingly healthy back experiences pain. Incidentally, the opposite is also true. Some backs look like they should be causing major problems: very curvy spines (hyper-lordosis, for example) or, even worse, very straight spines, sometimes cause surprisingly few problems to their owners and an embarrassing absence of explanation from therapists.

Pain is, after all, a "brain thing" and even with the latest imaging technology the most powerful high-resolution brain scans are not helpful if we do not know what to make of such images.

The bad news therefore is that this book will not attempt to help you identify the reason for your back pain.

Nor is it a manual for a new therapy or an illustrated exercise book offering 10 super-efficient back pain relief exercises. Books of this nature have been flooding the market for decades while the percentage of the population experiencing back pain, quite oblivious to the newest and most effective exercise ever conceived by marketing geniuses, has stagnated or grown in most countries.

What we need is a systemic approach. While many health experts claim to have a holistic approach, this is usually not true. Holistic or systemic approaches need to take into account everything that has any influence on a person. Sometimes, dysfunctional calf muscles can cause lower back pain and a therapist who considers this possibility might already be doing an above average job at helping his or her patient. Maybe he or she also takes nutrition into account.

But furniture, for example, is often forgotten, and so are clothes. A truly systemic approach must take a patient's car seat, office chair, shoes, mattress and belt into account, because all these things directly influence posture and tension in the body.

What good is doing one hour of sports a day to fight back pain, if the person spends another seven hours in poor sitting posture, wears shoes that damage the back for ten hours, and then goes to sleep on a mattress that encourages slouching for another eight hours?

Instead of trying quick fixes or one-exercise-fits-all solutions, this book is your guide to identifying and eliminating everything and anything from shoes, clothes and chairs, to ideas and habits, which stop your back from healing every day.

Because your body is constantly trying to heal itself. That's what it is programmed to do. Give it a chance.

THE STORY OF YOU

Before we move on, please take a good look at your biceps. Flex them, relax them, and admire them. Your biceps today are of course the result of how you have used them in the past. Whether you are a dedicated body-builder, a climber, a desk-worker or a couch potato, the way you use your body strongly influences what you make of your genetic capital.

This is true for the whole body. Your body is the story of how you have treated it along the road. It tells you a lot about genetics, but also about nutrition and exercise.

The central thesis of this book is that your back pains are either caused, or at least aggravated, by the way you use your body in everyday life.

And while your body is of course constantly trying to heal and eliminate the causes of back pain, the chances are that you are severely sabotaging the healing process. Sabotaging it enough, in many cases, to make your back pain chronic or permanent.

As I pointed out above, you very likely sleep in a bed that encourages bad posture. You probably wear shoes that put high strain on your lumbar region and neck. Your chair most likely either causes you to slump or weakens the muscles in your back. And even if it did enable you to develop good sitting posture, you may have no idea how to sit "properly".

All these little habits combined add up to almost twenty-four hours a day of bad influence. You are, so to speak, not only sleeping with the enemy, but also walking with it and sitting on it.

This is why, as long as you have not taken any action to deal with these everyday health risks, doing a bit of physiotherapy to cure your back is absolutely pointless. You exist twenty-four hours a day, 156 hours per week; a few hours of sport each week is nothing but a drop in the ocean.

Taking another step forward is fine - this book is about how to stop taking twenty-three steps back the rest of the day.

DOCTORS AND ELEPHANTS

If your back hurts badly or repeatedly you must of course see a doctor. No book or method can ever replace your GP's opinion and some conditions, be it kidney stones or a slipped disk, which lead to back pain, are frankly too dangerous to be left alone.

This does not mean that the doctor will have to operate. In fact, a German study conducted in Düsseldorf has recently shown that about half of all back operations were useless - to the patients that is. While it never hurts to get a second opinion you must ultimately trust your doctor's opinion and follow the advice given.

However, it could be argued that people who study medicine are not so much specialists in health, but rather, in sickness. Medical studies and training obviously focus on curing medical conditions much more than on how to preserve one's health.

Health, vibrant health, is much more than the mere absence of pains and ailments. Being truly healthy means having energy and being able to use your body to do whatever you enjoy. Healthy people feel strong and balanced and they take pleasure in using their bodies, be it for sports, sex, or just every day work-related activities.

I have a personal rule: You can't help someone with something that you can't get right yourself. If you are overweight, don't be a weight-loss coach. If you smoke, don't teach others how to quit smoking. If you have constant back-pain, take care of yourself before you try to "cure" others.

If this rule makes sense to you, you might want to choose your doctor or health-professional wisely. Knowing about sickness is not the same job as knowing about health. This is why a therapist in alternative medicine or a coach can play an important part in helping you to be truly healthy.

You also want your doctor to be honest with you to the point of bluntness. If there is an elephant in the room, they must be sure to point it out to you.

For example, are you overweight? Political correctness might keep your doctor or therapist from pointing out to you that being overweight will often cause or at least aggravate back pain.

Especially in men, the weight of a big stomach puts immense pressure on your lower back. Of course, life is unfair: while some people can devour entire plates the size of cartwheels of fried food and never put on a kilo, for some just reading this sentence is all it takes to gain weight.

Addressing the weight issue therefore should never be about making someone feel guilty or bad. It does not matter whether you are overweight mostly because of genetics or because of really bad eating habits. If you are overweight, then losing weight will almost always alleviate your back pain, alongside many other health benefits.

In case of doubt, please ask your doctor for advice on this matter. The media in particular distorts our perception of body image. You do not have to have the figure of Gwyneth Paltrow, but you should avoid that of Richard Griffiths, the wonderful actor who plays Uncle Vernon in the Harry Potter films.

Being overweight is not the only elephant in the room (no pun intended!). Maybe you are also a couch potato. If you drive to work, sit at a computer all day long, come home to dinner and an evening in front of the telly every day of the week and spend your weekends lying around, then look no further for now. Some of the nerves, especially in your lower back, will react to inactivity and start causing pain. And while there might be other causes, you won't know until you start getting a daily dose of back-friendly activity.

However, some people have the exact opposite problem. If you run a marathon every day or if you are a professional mover, roof tiler or do any other job that includes heavy lifting, maybe you overexert yourself every day. If your body does not get enough rest, it will obviously stop functioning well at some point.

It comes as a surprise to many patients that smoking also seems to cause back pain. As it lowers the amount of oxygen in the blood, smoking may cause disc degeneration from malnutrition. Correlations between smoking and herniation or disc height reduction have also been found.

INFLAMMATORY VS. MECHANICAL BACK PAIN

While this book concentrates on the mechanical aspect of back pain, inflamed tissue is an oft-neglected cause of back pain and must be diagnosed.

But how do you know whether you suffer from inflammatory or mechanical back pain? As a rule of thumb, if you suffer particularly after periods of immobility, especially at night and in the early morning, your tissue might be inflamed and you should consider this a possible cause that needs to be investigated.

This rule of thumb is not fool-proof, however, since sitting is an immobile position for most people and this induces mechanically caused back pain.

However, if you consider that your back pain might be caused by inflammation, see a doctor about the possibility of a prescription for anti-inflammatory drugs (NSAIDs) and be particularly vigilant about your diet.

I still suggest that you follow the recommendations in this book just the same, because there is no point in making things worse and we are yet to fully determine the extent to which mechanical and inflammatory back pain are interdependent.

STRESS

While I am no fan of esoteric or unproven theories, the link between psychology and back pain is, at the very least, an anecdotal truth. Though the exact causality of stress-related back pain may never be proven, it is an established fact that good mood allows for a higher tolerance to pain while bad mood has the opposite effect. Regardless of whether or not you believe that stress and a bad mood can cause back pain, you can safely assume they are making it worse.

Such conditions therefore have to be addressed and treated. They are also invisible elephants if you don't point them out to your therapist, so ensure you give him or her all the information that might help solve the puzzle.

TLDR (TOO LONG, DIDN'T READ)

Your body has the natural ability to heal itself and recover - be it from the flu or a cut from a kitchen knife. Bad posture may not always be the only cause of chronic back pain, but it will always stand in the way of the back getting better.

Even the best tools, if used the wrong way, will break. Your body in general and your back in particular make no exception to this rule. The key to fighting back pain often lies not so much in adopting new habits (like sports or massage) but in identifying and eliminating the habits that caused the problem in the first place. Such habits relate to posture, but also unhealthy shoes or mattresses. There is little point taking one step forward if you have to stop and take 23 back.

1
SLEEPING WITH THE ENEMY

A laugh and a long sleep are the best cures for everything.

Irish Proverb

How a soft mattress reinforces your hunchback and makes you nervous. The difference between body-structure and posture. The importance of connective tissue.

THE MISSING LINK: CONNECTIVE TISSUE (FASCIA)

Doctors and cooks share a traditional disregard for connective tissue. Anatomy classes basically consist of cutting it away, so that students can learn about the origins and insertions (the ends) of muscles and see which bones they attach to.

If you sometimes cook meat, depending on the cut you choose, you might notice different "compartments" of a muscle or a group of muscles, separated by a thin white film. Often, this film will get thicker towards the end; this is when we call it a tendon. Tendons are very resistant and hard to chew, that is why we also cut them out and leave the connective tissue.

Unless you are in desperate need of a bowstring, the connective tissue of a dead animal is often of little use.

However, when trying to understand about musculoskeletal pain in general, or back pain in particular, connective tissue is often the missing link without which we cannot satisfactorily understand posture, body structure and movement.

Connective tissue, as the words suggest, connects things. As a matter of fact, it connects everything in the body. It is found around your bones, inner organs and, of course, muscles, like cling film around a portion of ground meat. If you twist the ends of your cling film, it becomes thicker and stronger. This is when we call it tendon and it is therefore actually this tendon, or fascia, not the muscle itself, that connects to the bone. Movement therefore is not just muscle and bone. It's muscle, connective tissue, also called fascia, and bone.

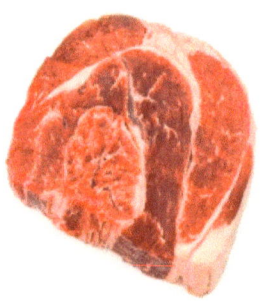

Figure 1.1
This beef shin beautifully shows how the fascia (white film-like tissue) surrounds different muscles.

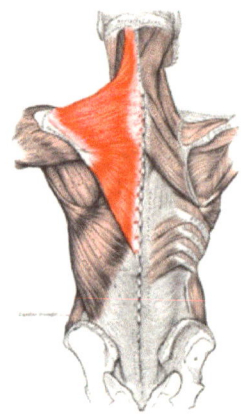

Figure 1.2
The trapezius muscle.

But your fascia plays other important roles in your well-being. If you cut through a piece of beef shin you will find that different muscles often lie on top of, or right next to, one another (Figure 1.1).

Fascia separates these muscles and allows them to work independently. To enable this there is a constant flow of lymph between the different muscles that allows for frictionless movement

22

of the different parts, the same way oil aids movement in a motor. Or at least, that's how it should be. In some cases the lymph can locally dry out, rendering independent movement of adjacent muscles difficult or impossible.

You will learn many other fascinating facts about fascia later on in this book, but, in order to understand why mattresses matter, you do need to know that fascia are highly malleable and, whilst they shape the body, they are themselves shaped by the use we make of them.

In simple terms, a sheath of connective tissue consists of two elements, which vary in proportion according to how the tissue is used. One component is the highly elastic elastin; the other one is the sturdier collagen. While collagen is the main protein and gives your tissue strength, the amount of elastin determines how flexible and stretchable the tissue is. Imagine the difference between a piece of string and a strong rubber band.

The difference is very visible in people's shoulders and in the state of their trapezius muscle in particular. The trapezius is a triangular muscle that connects the base of your skull to your shoulder blade and your spine (Figure 1.2)[2].

In some people, this muscle is nicely relaxed at most times and hardly visible, while in older people or people who often carry bags on their shoulders or do body-building, the muscle is constantly under tension and lifting up the shoulder.

In fact, most people lose the capacity to fully relax their shoulders as soon as they reach their twenties. You can easily tell if this is

---

2   For the purposes of illustrating this point, we are only talking about the superior part of this muscle.

the case by looking at the angle of their collarbones. If they are perfectly horizontal, their shoulder is truly relaxed. However, from personal experience I estimate that not more than one in ten adults still has truly relaxed and functional shoulders.

In a neutral position, your shoulders should neither be pulled forwards by your pectoris muscles, nor backwards by your trapezius and rhomboid muscles, but be positioned in the middle.

However, misuse of the shoulder in every day life often leads to a shoulder whose default position is no longer vertically and horizontally neutral, but often permanently lifted upwards and pulled forwards. This is often the result of pulling the shoulder forward for writing and typing and upward for carrying a handbag and lifting a glass or a fork (Figure 1.3).

Constantly holding the shoulder in an up-forwards position will lead the connective tissue to adapt and modify. This is how, through permanent misuse, bad posture becomes bad body-structure. Especially carrying heavy bags on one shoulder will lead the tissue to change and augment the percentage of collagen fibers. The shoulder will become capable of maintaining the elevated position for longer, but will lose some of its flexibility and range of movement as a result.

Now imagine a person with a hunchback. Not quite the hunchback of Notre Dame, necessarily, but any position where the head is no longer resting on the shoulders but carried in front of them. The head-torso relationship is an easy way to know whether you have good posture. If you look at children and young people and those lucky enough to still have good posture after the age of twenty, the center of gravity of the skull is situated exactly over the shoulders most of the time.

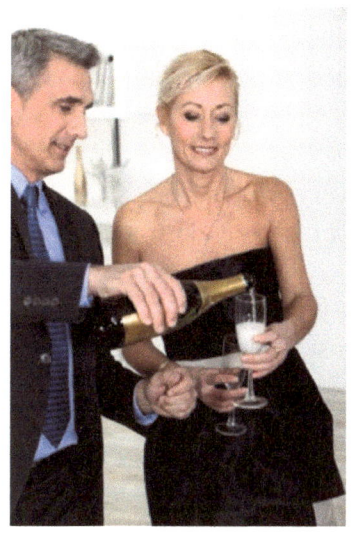

Figure 1.3

This is a good example of dysfunctional shoulders in adults. In order to hold the glasses, the woman lifts up her shoulders with a very visible trapezius muscle. Also, note how she pulls the shoulders forwards. This results in a sunken chest and Head-Forward-Posture.

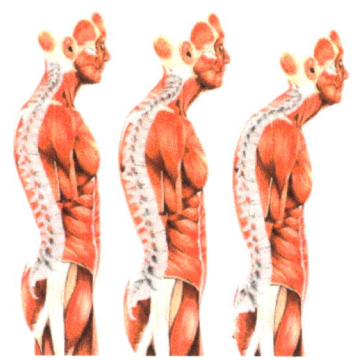

Figure 1.4

The Head-Forward-Posture often starts evolving in the early twenties. The neck muscles now have to carry the head instead of balancing it out and the lever effect adds to the immense amount of work these muscles now have to provide.

Also, note how the sternum is automatically pushed inwards as the head goes forward. This makes deep and relaxed breathing near impossible.

Thus, the neck and shoulder muscles have to balance, but not carry the head. However, as we develop a rounded back, the head starts moving forwards and its entire weight has to be held by constantly tensed neck muscles (Figure 1.4).

Mechanically, as the head goes forward, the sternum goes in and the back becomes rounded. Thus, in the same way that the center of gravity of the head is no longer directly on top of the shoulders, the center of gravity of the entire torso is no longer situated above but rather, in front of, the pelvis. This creates a lever effect on the junction between your pelvis and your torso, which is your lower back, the lumbar region.

While your lower back is perfectly capable of supporting the weight of the torso situated above it, a prolonged or permanent strain can be harmful for the structure.

If you have a slightly rounded back in every day life, your connective tissue will adapt to this posture and fix or bind you to it, just like in the case of the shoulder.

This is how posture, the way you are positioned in space at a given moment, becomes body-structure. Body structure is the general form of your body. While your posture changes all the time, your structure evolves - or deteriorates - slowly. You could say that structure is your default posture, the position in space your body has when "it is doing nothing".

In summary, we all develop our own personal body structure according to the way we use our body. Imagine your connective tissue as an endless net that stretches through the whole body. It wraps and connects bones, muscle and organs. Body structure is the sum of tensions in the connective tissue that deform us ever so slightly, but permanently, to give us our unique shape.

See this child's toy that consists of rubber connections and sticks, just like bones and tendons (Figure 1.5). Its form is ultimately determined by the tension in the rubber bands.

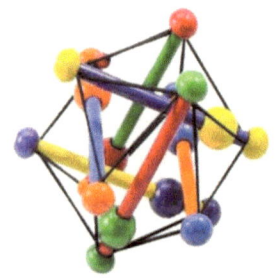

Figure 1.5

This toy obtains its form from the tension of the rubber bands and the stiffness of the "bones". It is an example of Tensegrity – a term coined by famous architect Richard Buckminster Fuller.

If one of the bands is looser or tighter than usual, the whole structure takes a different shape. This is why holistic therapy, which treats the body as a whole, will sometimes work on your leg to treat your bad back. Simply because it may be one of the muscles in your leg that is too tense that is pulling your pelvis into a bad position.

SOFT OR FIRM – THE OLD MATTRESS CONUNDRUM

People sleep an average of about one third of their lives or eight hours a day. Also, sleeping time is healing time, which makes your sleeping habits even more important for your well-being. Unfortunately, the erroneous idea that a soft bed is a comfortable bed and that you should have a pillow nicely propped under your head persists. Therefore, many people reinforce the bad posture they have in the daytime at night too. They take eight steps back instead of forwards.

Gravity and a hard mattress combined can give you a good posture workout at night if you only let them. I will explain this in the next section, when I go through different sleeping positions. The point I want to make relates to the anatomical and physical.

Those who do convert to harder mattresses often experience an unexpected side benefit. They sleep deeper and move less at night. On a futon, you might even find yourself waking up in the very position you first went to sleep in.

This side effect is not just mechanical, it relates to your nervous system, which naturally obsesses over balance and stability. To understand the benefit of a hard mattress, try standing on one foot on a soft mattress or sofa. Be careful not to fall and hurt yourself!

Now try standing on a wooden floor, again on one foot. You will find that the latter is much easier and lets you relax much more than the former - because *stability comes from resistance*. The harder the floor, the better it supports your weight and the more efficient the little movements you make to keep in balance.

When you are lying down, a hard surface will provide the same kind of exact and reassuring feedback to your brain. This feedback tells your brain that you are stable, and not, as it were, rolling out of your cave or falling from the tree. Little things like this used to be major survival traits.

That is why a futon is reassuring for your nervous system, while a soft water bed will only confuse it.

If you pay attention to just how relaxed you can keep the rest of your body when standing on the hard floor, compared to trying to find your balance on a soft surface, you will see a big difference.

In the same way, your body will not be able to fully relax on a soft surface. The extra tension in the muscles is called stress and is not conducive to a good night's relaxing sleep.

SLEEPING ON YOUR BACK

Most people tend to develop a rounded back and rounded shoulders over time. Especially in the daytime, bad chairs, our shoes, and poor sitting posture encourage this hunchback posture. Now imagine someone with a hunchback going to sleep on his or her back on a soft mattress.

The person will simply sink into the mattress because the mattress is soft and unable to offer any resistance, so the rounded back and convex posture will remain exactly the same (Figure 1.6). Most people make things even worse by putting their head on a plump pillow. Now imagine the posture of a person lying on a soft mattress with a pillow under their head. Mentally turn that picture by ninety degrees and you can see they are simply in a horizontal hunchback of Notre Dame position (Figure 1.8 left).

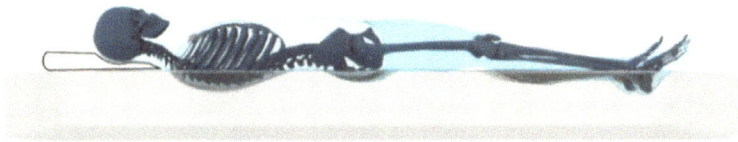

Figure 1.6

Hunchback during the day and a hunchback at night: A soft mattress and a pillow will encourage a slouching position even at night. Staying for an additional eight hours with a round back and forward neck and shoulders will make your posture permanent. This will become your body structure. When you mentally turn that sleeping posture by ninety degrees, it becomes even more visible just how harmful this is.

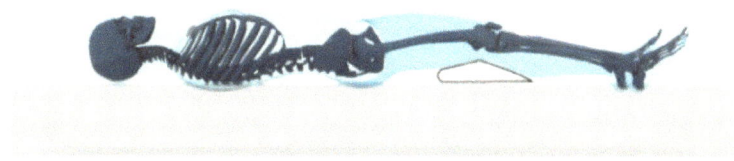

Figure 1.7

A hard mattress achieves the opposite effect. Gravity pulls rounded shoulders back and a rounded back down into a straight position all night. Without a pillow, the head will also position itself on top of the torso. The pillow under the knees will provide lower back pain relief.

On a hard mattress like a futon for example, things work out quite differently. Without the aid of a soft mattress that allows you to sink in, the convex shape of a round back would be pulled into a much flatter, straighter position by gravity. With a very flat or no pillow under your head, you get a free, all-night posture stretch, courtesy of your old friend, gravity. Mentally turn the picture in your mind again and there you see a person with good posture (Figure 1.8 right).

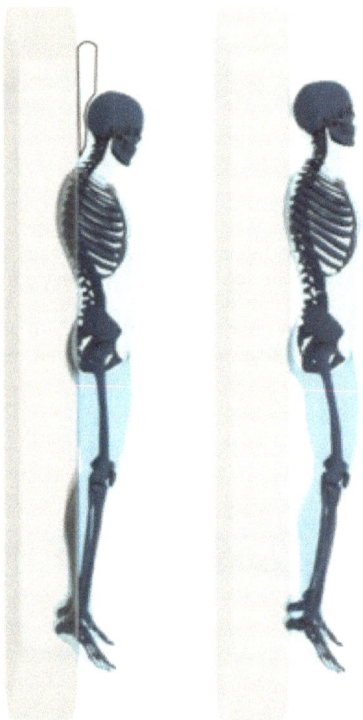

Figure 1.8

How small changes make a big difference in the long run. By turning the sleeping postures by 90°, you can see what a big difference there is between soft and hard mattresses.

The pillow that you have no further use for under your head should be placed under your knees. This creates further relaxation for your lower back. Some people with lower back problems may actually find bending their knees mandatory in order to find some relief for their lower back. They should also do an exercise[3] explained on my YouTube channel to relax the lower back when lying down.

This is of course an unpopular view if you are in the mattress business, because making a simple hard mattress is rather easy and then what will you sell people? How can you sell special springs or memory foam or anything that makes your mattress expensive?

SLEEPING ON YOUR SIDE

Of course, we often see pictures of people sleeping on their sides and hear the argument that their spine needs support in order to stay straight.

A very simple test lets you verify this assertion. Lie down on your side on a hard floor and make sure your neck is sufficiently supported. This time of course you do need a pillow. To support your neck, or cervical vertebrae, the pillow should be as thick as your shoulder is wide.

This is probably where you find out just how useless your pillow is. While it's probably too thick to put your head on it when lying on your back, it's probably nowhere near thick enough to support it when lying on your side.

Anyway, now that you have stabilized your head, let's find out if your spine needs special support to stay straight. How much force

---

3 https://youtu.be/MjpHQq2yd10

do you actually need to keep a straight spine in the side position? The answer is of course none at all, which is also how much use you have for a special mattress for your back.

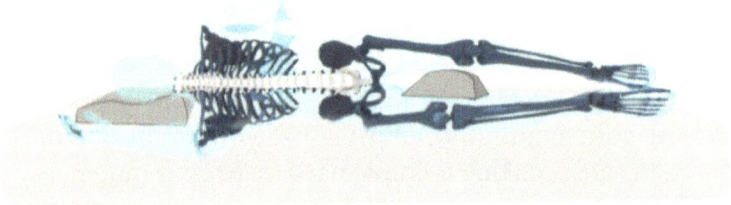

Figure 1.9
When sleeping on your side, make sure to use a firm pillow, keeping your head in line with the spine. A pillow between the knees will most often relax your lower back too.

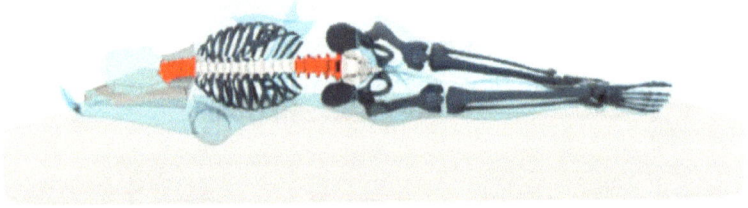

Figure 1.10
Lying on your side with a soft pillow will strain your neck at night. Especially if you have wider hipbones, a pillow between the knees might be essential.

If you are a side sleeper, don't throw away your useless pillow, you might find it relaxing to put it between your knees (Figure 1.9).

Sleeping on your side is second best to sleeping on your back. Women can experience some discomfort on very hard mattress if the top of the thighbone (femur) does not have sufficient "padding". Very wide hips can also create a problem when combined with narrow shoulders, but this is only problematic in a few individuals.

In any case, a lot of body weight rests on one shoulder when sleeping on the side. This should be avoided, especially in case of shoulder and neck pain.

As a caveat, some people have medical conditions that require them to sleep in special beds. If this is your case, please disregard these general explanations and follow your doctor's advice.

SLEEPING ON YOUR FRONT

I will not go further into the ventral (stomach) sleeping position, as you should try to avoid it on principle because it invariably puts strain on your neck. However, if this is the only position in which you feel you can go to sleep, you can try putting a pillow under your pelvis and under your ankles.

A person changing a soft for a harder mattress will often experience sore muscles in the beginning. This is actually a good sign, it's the result of the workout gravity has given you in your sleep and an eight hour workout can be quite a challenge in the beginning. Especially because the rounder your back, the more of a workout your tissue gets. Sometimes a more gradual change can constitute a better, i.e. more sustainable, strategy here.

TLDR

Connective tissue adapts to poor posture and creates a more permanent bad body structure. This structure consists mostly of a hunched back and a head that is too far in front of the body.

A soft mattress will support this convex body shape when sleeping on one's back and maintain this bad posture for the whole night, thus contributing to a vicious circle. A thick pillow under your neck will make things even worse, by pushing your head even further in front of your shoulders.

On a hard mattress, gravity will pull the body down and stretch it back into a straighter, more natural posture all night. With no pillow, or just a very flat one, your head will also resume its natural place on top of the shoulders, thus relaxing the neck muscles.

Furthermore, a hard mattress offers better stability to the body, thus allowing the nervous system to know where it is in space and to be reassured that you will not fall out of bed (or from your tree or out of your cave!). This reassurance is essential in allowing the nervous system to lower overall levels of tension, which in turn results in a deeper, more relaxed sleep.

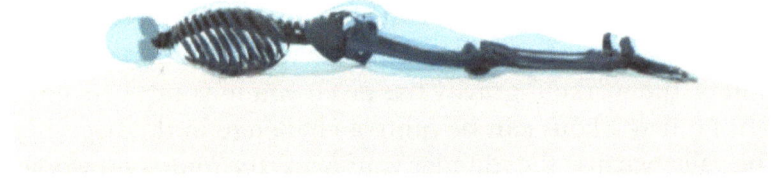

Figure 1.11
Sleeping on your front puts a lot of strain on your neck and should be avoided.

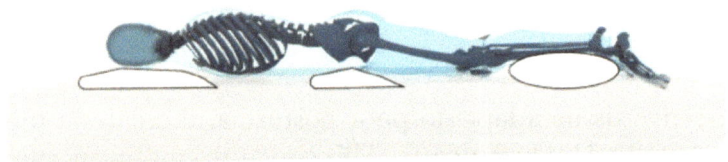

Figure 1.12
Positioning a pillow under your pelvis and ankles will allow for more relaxed calf muscles and reduce tension in you lower back. Another pillow under your sternum might also alleviate neck problems, if only slightly.

2
TRY WALKING IN THESE SHOES

I have two doctors, my left leg and my right.

G.M. Trevelyan

Introducing the ZigZag-Line principle. How shoes determine your whole posture. Why even low heels are detrimental to your health. More problems created by shoes.

THE ZIGZAG LINE PRINCIPLE

Of course size matters; height certainly seems to, anyway. Introduced by European nobility in the 18th century, heels were first worn by men at court. Women rapidly adopted the fashion and it is today still the norm to buy shoes with heels.

From extravagant 18-centimeter stilettos to the fifteen-millimeter heels on men's business shoes, shoemakers persist in showing off their fashion sense while demonstrating their total lack of awareness in health matters.

To understand why heels are so harmful, you need to first understand how to stand properly. If you look at the profile of a human skeleton and its joints, someone with good posture will look a bit like an accordion. If you imagine a vertical centerline through the body, very much like the wick in a candle, you realize that the ankles and pelvis are slightly behind this line, while the knees and the center of gravity of the torso are ever so slightly in front of it. The head rests in the very center of this line. This makes sense, when you consider which muscles are supposed to keep a body upright: the calves, the thigh muscles, the buttocks and the muscles along the spine. These are the muscles designed to open joints and to push the body up.

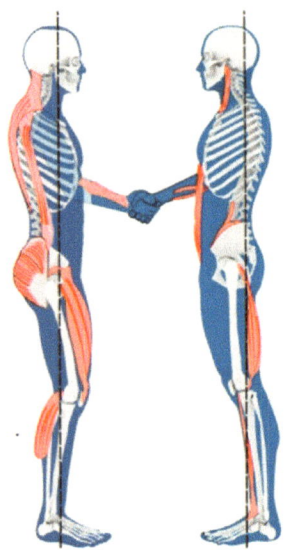

Figure 2.1

Small changes can make a big difference: The person on the left hand side is standing correctly in the zigzag line position, while the person on the right hand side over-extends his knees. This results in a pelvis and head that are pushed forwards, resulting in pain.

When a person stands barefoot in this slight zigzag line, their joints are perfectly aligned to let these muscles resist gravity and keep us upright. The angle of the pelvis and the rib cage allow the organs to have room to function.

When a person suffers from a hunchback, often combined with a Head-Forward-Posture and overstretched knees, this changes not only the position of the joints, but also which muscles the person uses to keep upright.

The antagonists of the muscles that should allow us to stand upright are the muscles that close joints, such as the hamstrings, the *psoas-illiacus* (which bends the hip) and the six-pack, the straight stomach muscles.

One typical bad posture results from overstretched knees and a pelvis that is too far in front of the body. This is a typically male posture and you can also recognize it by the fact that when walking or standing, a person with this type of body structure usually has both feet pointing outwards, a bit like Charlie Chaplin.

In this case, it is not the muscles in your back, but your stomach muscles and mainly the rectus *abdominis* that keeps your torso up. As you already know, a tense rectus *abdominis* will keep you from breathing; but this is just one of many reasons why you should use flexor muscles to keep you upright.

In a major case of a hunchback, while the designated muscles in your back do have to do the assigned work of keeping you upright, the lever effect of your body weight is such that these muscles now have to do much more work than they are designed for.[4]

In architecture, statics is the science of how a building stands up and resists gravity. The human body faces the same challenge and has to obey the same physical laws.

---

4   I hope Richard Dawkins and Charles Darwin will forgive me for using this intellectual shortcut and I assure the reader that I am aware that we weren't "designed" but have evolved into our current form.

HOW HEELS DISRUPT NATURAL BODY-ALIGNMENT

In geometry, three points determine a surface. This is why a table with three legs will be stable on almost any surface. If it had only two legs, it would tend to fall over. A table with four legs might not fall over but it will wobble if it stands on an uneven surface.

The human foot has indeed three points of contact with the ground: The heel and the two pads, the one outside behind the little toe and the other inside, behind the big toe, that touch the horizontal surface we stand on (Figure 2.2). When we stand like this, our vertical wick-line is perfectly angled at 90° with the floor.

Relative to our height, the surface on which we stand is very small - we are in fact skyscrapers, not bungalows. Now imagine if a skyscraper were to be built on the side of a hill or a mountain without flattening the ground. You would get a second leaning tower of Pisa - but not for very long.

Because of the relative height of a human body, we experience the very same problem. A heel changes the angle of the surface you stand on. If you are 180 cm tall and the distance between your heel and your forefoot is fifteen centimeters, the top of your head would be moved 15 centimeters forward by heels only one centimeter high.

In the same way, if you are only 160 cm tall, have smaller feet (10 cm length from heel to foot pads) but wear 4 cm heels, the bigger angle would push you forward by an incredible 64 cm at your highest point (Figure 2.4). But only if you keep your body in the aforementioned perfect upright position along the ZigZag-Line. Which of course you cannot do, because you would simply fall over.

What actually happens is that your body compensates for the unnatural angle of your foot, sometimes by pushing the pelvis forward and adopting a rounder back posture, more often by using the back muscles to over-extend the spine. This looks like good posture but is a major strain on both the discs and the muscles and will invariably end in pain - if only from exhaustion.

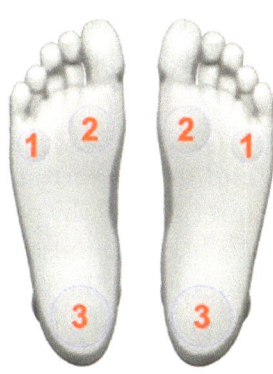

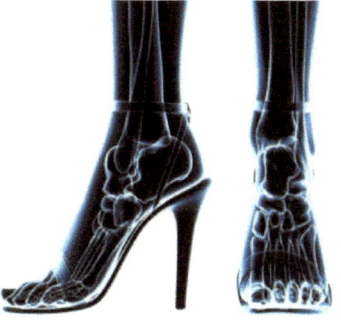

Figure 2.2

There are three points of contact between your feet and the ground. Arches link these points.

Figure 2.3

High heels put a lot of strain on your foot. They also cause bunions and back pain. One therefore has to choose between beautiful shoes and beautiful feet.

It is therefore particularly ironic that some people offer courses on how to have good posture in high heels. This is along the same line as *The Role of Arsenic in a Healthy Diet.*

High heels wouldn't be a problem if we only wore them occasionally. The body can adapt to different circumstances without sustaining major long-term damage. But what happens when we stand at an angle ten hours a day, every day of the year?

Well, it deforms not only your feet (Figure 2.3), but also your entire body. Your pelvis, which is formed like a deep bowl, is designed to accommodate and give room to your digestive system and reproductive organs. Like any part of the body or organ, the whole business works best when everything is in its rightful place, i.e. "in the pelvis". When tilted too far forward or backwards for a longer amount of time, the whole plumbing system gets squashed and is therefore prone to functioning less efficiently.

In the very same way, you already know that a round back pushes the shoulders forward and the sternum in. The sternum thus encroaches on the room needed for your stomach and heart. Again, not advisable.

With time, as always, the body adapts and the "deformity" it takes on becomes one's own personal posture. This is why people sometimes experience different side effects like sore muscles or back pain when they start walking in flat shoes again. But just like with proper mattresses, this is mostly just a transitional phase and shows to what extent the body has become used to being crooked.

From my experience as a therapist, I have observed just how much harm bad shoes do to people every day. People, especially women, often don't even realize how contradictory it is to wear heels to work every day, but then pursue massage or sport as a way of getting rid of their back pain.

If you are someone who has good proprioception (a feeling for your body) and are used to healthy shoes, you immediately notice just how harmful even low heels are to your balance.

What is particularly interesting here, is that not only lifestyle magazines, but often even health professionals proclaim how "small heels are good to support (or relieve) the back".

When hearing assertions like these, it is always fun to ask simple questions. So, if slight heels are good for your back, then, presumably, being barefoot isn't? Hmmm…

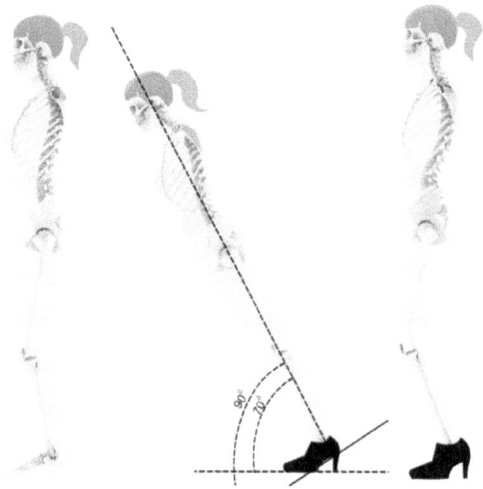

Figure 2.4

There is a 90° angle between your feet and the ground. When standing correctly and naturally, this allows for perfect body alignment. Heels artificially lift up the heel, while the forefoot stays in contact with the ground. This creates an unnatural angle, for which the body will have to compensate in order not to lose balance. This leads to higher pressure in the lower back and an overstretched spine.

Even if we accept that heels might be good in some cases, how do we then calculate the right height? Which formula tells us that 2mm might be too little, but 4cm too much of a heel? How does the formula change with each person, what are the variables?

Also, how come after thousands of years of evolution we now need heels to make a fully functioning human body?

To be very blunt I believe that a therapist (not a doctor, they do other things) or a posture expert who wears heels (or sneakers) has not even started thinking about good posture in every day life. Wearing heels just doesn't make any sense in relation to good posture.

Before I finish this paragraph on heels, I would like to suggest a little exercise to show you how something that seemingly only happens in your ankle does in fact affect the whole body.

Exercise:

Make sure you are barefoot and lay a book on the floor (thickness roughly two centimeters). First, stand next to the book, in an upright relaxed position, your head straight and the eyes looking straight to the horizon. Slowly open and close your mouth and feel exactly where your upper and lower teeth touch.

Then, repeat the exercise, but with your heels resting on the book, as if you were wearing shoes. Again, close your mouth and compare where the teeth touch.

Try it right now.

Yes, even though both positions allow you to look straight forward and have your skull at the same angle, the overall statics of the body have changed and not even your jaw functions the same way. Now think of the difference this makes in your spine or to the angle of your pelvis.

If you are not too shy, you could do this exercise in underwear and take pictures of your profile. Compare the shape of the spine or the length and angle of your neck. You will be amazed.

If only the bad news about shoes stopped there. Unfortunately, we are only just getting started.

KERS - THE FORMULA ONE TECHNOLOGY IN YOUR FEET

Someone had a great idea in Formula One. What if they could store some of the energy from braking and put it back into acceleration? The Kinetic Energy Recovery System (KERS) does just this: It momentarily stores the vehicle's kinetic energy from braking for later use in acceleration. This can be done mechanically using a flywheel or electrically with a capacitor. There is no need to go into the mechanical details here, but did you know that your feet (and calves) were designed to act as mechanical KERS? It's too bad that most shoes do not allow for this wonderful mechanism to function.

If you are still barefoot, do the following. Place your foot on a sheet of paper and trace its shape with a pencil. When you have done this, fetch the shoes you wear most often, put them on the same sheet and trace the shape again. This makes many people laugh, especially women or Italian businessmen. Because there are few items of clothing so obviously not shaped to fit a human body.

Your feet, as you can probably see, get wider towards the toes, whereas most shoes are pointy. Yes, if shoemakers applied their genius to motorcycle helmets we would have heads shaped like pyramids. *"Well, who cares?"* they might say, *"it looks good, doesn't it?"*

But wearing shoes conceived for aliens does not only bring about pain. If you look at your feet, you see 26 little bones and lots of muscle and connective tissue (Figure 2.5). This is particularly useful in a foot because it allows it to absorb, store and release kinetic energy:

Just like a very tight rubber band, your connective tissue is elastic. When pulled apart, it can store energy just like a rubber band.

The three pads you stand on are connected by arches: The main one on the inside, a flatter, but nonetheless important one on the outside, and a third one between the inner and outer pad. When you transfer the weight of your body onto your foot, this construction of bones and tissue will absorb part of the energy in the connective tissue (Figure 2.6). The arches will flatten and the tissue in the foot and the Achilles tendon tenses. As you go forward, this kinetic energy is then released.[5]

You can try this out for yourself by observing how your foot slightly spreads out when you make a little jump forward and land on one leg.

Imagine someone dribbling a ball. Every time it touches the ground, it will deform ever so slightly and this energy will push it back up. If it cannot deform because it is too hard, it will probably break or crack, like glass. If it is very soft, like a ball made of foam, it will mostly absorb the energy and bounce very little.

This is why you should always try walking in new shoes or even running a bit. Because only then will you know whether the shoe is in fact wide enough for your foot to flatten out. Because if it isn't, not only will your foot constantly hurt itself against the shoe and your walk become less efficient, but your tissue will lose its springy quality and the ability to absorb energy. A bit like wearing ski boots instead of slippers.

---

5   You can find more information on the human KERS system in my YouTube video here: https://www.youtube.com/watch?v=JJZk3PB5Ulg

As people get older they are more and more frightened of falling as it becomes harder and harder for them to maintain good balance.

When you stand on one foot you can feel all the slight muscle movement your brain has to ask your lower leg and foot to perform in order to keep your balance. Of course, if your leg and foot have been in a cast for weeks or in tight shoes for decades, the

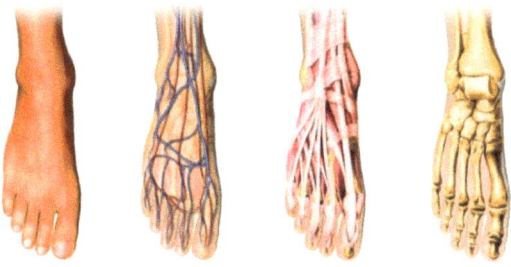

Figure 2.5

The human foot is a beautiful complex construction of muscle, bones and connective tissue. It's a natural shock absorber which does not need any help from the shoe industry and will do its job perfectly unless restricted and made useless in tight shoes with thick soles.

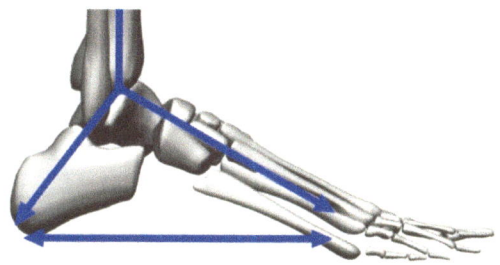

Figure 2.6

Every step is a small fall. If your heels touch the ground first, the shock cannot be absorbed. However, by touching with the forefoot first, the arches of the foot will widen and absorb the energy. This energy will then push you forward and help you with the next step. This is how one can achieve an efficient and natural gait.

resulting atrophy will make these little adjustments much harder. Thus, a healthy and flexible foot does not only allow for a pain-free, efficient walk, it also helps you keep your balance and avoid falling in the future.

In general, you should also avoid lacing a shoe too tightly, which makes things even worse.

HOW YOUR SHOES MAKE YOU "BLIND"

British author Douglas Adams famously equipped one of his characters with "coolness sunglasses". In dangerous situations, these glasses turn completely dark thus allowing you to keep an admiringly cool attitude to oncoming danger.

Your retina hosts more than a hundred million receptors called rods and cones that let you see your environment. How much of your natural resolution are you willing to give up?

This is obviously a silly question, we'd all like to have and maintain perfect vision, which is, after all, a key survival trait. Especially so because vision, along with the inner ear and the feedback from your feet, helps the body keep in balance and avoid falling.

However, vision often declines with age, as does the quality of feedback coming from your inner ear.

Touch, haptic feedback, does not suffer the same rate of decline. Haptic feedback therefore becomes more and more important as you age.

Your feet are particularly good at this, with an estimated one hundred to two hundred thousand nerve endings per sole. These nerve endings can send very precise information about the ground you are standing on to your brain. The brain can then in turn analyze this information and make informed decisions about how to best keep the body in balance.

Unless, of course, you wear the shoe equivalent to coolness sunglasses! Shoes, that is, whose soles keep your nerve endings from feeling anything at all, by virtue of being so thick and/or hard that no information gets through at all.

This is the case in 99% of all shoes on the market. Their thick soles make you blind by preventing your nerve endings from gathering information about the ground you're standing on. Just imagine what this total absence of information from your feet does to the area of the brain that is designed to process it. Chances are, that area is probably not growing.

It is often argued that you need thick soles to protect your feet. You don't, not if you have healthy feet. Thin and flexible but resistant soles do a great job of protecting your feet and still letting them feel the ground at the same time.

Some shoes go even further in incapacitating your body. Not only do they act as a cast on your foot, but also on your ankle. This happens when your shoe is higher than your ankle and rather tight. Unless the weather makes it necessary, for the sake of a flexible foot and leg, you should always avoid shoes higher than your ankle. Boots impede natural ankle movement.

Of course, your ankles are probably not designed to handle the torque that they have to cope with when skiing. The situation is different when it comes to hiking though. Most hiking boots "protect" the ankle using sturdy leather and people tend to pull the laces rather tight to avoid spraining the ankle when walking.

I agree that this works, but then wouldn't it be safer to go hiking in a wheelchair to protect the knees and a neck brace to protect the neck?

It could be argued that this would slightly defeat the purpose of hiking… but that depends. If your only goal lies in getting from A to B, you are doing fine and are almost certain not to hurt your knees or neck. However, if your goal in hiking is also doing a healthy activity, why exclude your ankles from the party? While you supposedly train your whole body, why put the ankles in a cast?

If you impede the function of a major joint included in the walking process, can you really expect the whole movement to be remotely natural?

HOW TO BE YOUR OWN CHIROPRACTOR

And while we are on the subject of walking, did you know that walking right can be a formidable, extremely pleasant and efficient way of relaxing your lower back? So good, that you might never need a massage again?

Watch the way a cat walks. Its spine hangs like a washing line between its shoulders and its pelvis. Every step it takes twists and torques the spine by virtue of the counter movement between shoulders and pelvis. Because when the left front paw goes forward, so does the shoulder, but on the other end it is the right side of the pelvis that goes forward.

This counter-rotative movement is found in some techniques used by chiropractors and bonesetters and can be effective pain relief for humans. They will put you on a table; turn your torso one way and the pelvis and knees the other way. This will often result in an audible cracking sound in your lower back and then the spine feels lighter and relieved.

There is much debate on the long-term effectiveness and risk involved in using such techniques. But this is beside the point. The question should be why they are even necessary. Can bipeds not benefit from the natural spine movement in walking, exactly as quadrupeds do?

The answer is that they could, but in most cases don't because of their unnatural walking style. Walking can be your secret weapon against mechanical back pain if you are doing it right. It relaxes the back and brings life back into joints.

The problem starts with the fact that people have the completely wrong idea about the mechanics of walking.

Ask yourself which part of your foot is first to touch the ground when you walk?

For most people it's the heel. Actually, if you walk around barefoot and put your fingers in your ears, you might hear the thudding sound that your heel makes when it strikes the floor.

Why do you touch the ground with your heel first? This might seem like an unusual question - it's just what happens, isn't it? Well, think about which part of your foot touches first when you jog or run or jump. When you dance, box, go up and down the stairs or sneak into the children's bedroom to see whether they are successfully faking being asleep...

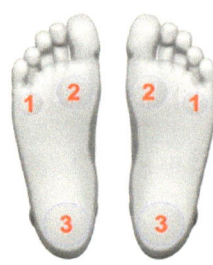

Figure 2.7

If your foot is relaxed, this is the order in which the balls of your feet should touch the ground - whether you are running, dancing, boxing or walking.

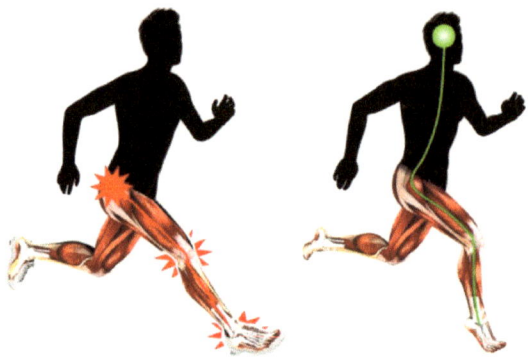

Figure 2.8

Only modern running shoes will allow you to touch the ground with your heels first. Whether you are walking or running, touching the ground with the heel first sends a shock wave through your ankles, knees, and pelvis. It is much healthier and more intelligent to touch the ground with the forefoot first. This allows for shock absorption, is much less abrasive for your joints and will let you transform the energy from impact into forward motion.

You probably touch the floor with your forefoot first in these situations. This should make you realize that, even for humans, the heel-strike, far from being the norm, is actually the exception. It is even more exceptional when you look at how your cat or dog walks, or indeed, every other animal. Do they lift up their paws and touch with their "heels" first when walking? No they don't.

Elephants seem to do it, but when you look at their actual bone structure, you realize that anatomy wouldn't allow it even if they tried.

This makes the human gait even more exceptional. Of course, we are different and bipedal, so let's get back to human anatomy.

Now some people will tell you that your heel touches the ground first so that you can "roll off from your heel to let your momentum carry you forward". This actual quote from an instructor video on Nordic Walking (yes, you can reverse thousands of years of evolution and go back to being a quadruped thanks to the ski-pole industry. Please applaud their marketing gurus for convincing people to buy ski poles in the summer) is utterly nonsensical.

First of all, have a close look at the anatomy of a foot. Things that roll, like car wheels, basketballs and a Camembert cheese have one thing in common: They are round. A quick look at Figure 2.6 however, reminds us of the fact that a human foot is not. It is not even convex, which would have been sufficient. The human foot is concave - it has arches. This simple fact tells us that wanting to roll off your heel is anatomical nonsense.

If you could roll off your heel and let the momentum carry you forward, you could, for example, make a big jump forward and land on your heels to test this. If you actually tried this, you would find out that while our "intelligent" neo-cortex might believe in such theoretical nonsense, our older and much wiser "reptile brain" will not allow you to actually attempt such a thing. It knows it wouldn't work and will force you to land correctly on your forefoot after all.

Lift up your leg and relax your ankle so that it is in a natural position. Now slowly and delicately lower your foot until it touches the floor. Don't move the ankle. It will turn out that the first thing to touch the ground will actually be the outside pad of your forefoot, the one right behind your small toe. This same place touches the ground first when you run or if you do rope jumping.

Therefore, all you have to do in order to achieve a natural walking movement is to avoid actively lifting your foot before it touches the ground. You know how to do this from sprinting and jogging. Thus, by doing less, your gait will become much more natural and the outside of your forefoot will touch the ground first. The tissue in your feet and the Achilles tendon will act as a shock absorber and stretch a little before releasing their tension as your body goes forward and transforming the absorbed energy into forward motion.

One more thing for those who find it difficult to let go of the mental picture of a rolling foot. When a human being walks, they constantly bend and straighten the knees. In fact, our muscles in general and those in our legs in particular, cannot push our body forward. They can only push it upwards and downwards by stretching and bending the ankles, knees and the pelvis. Therefore the center of gravity naturally goes up and down. The energy potential that the body has to make use of is therefore mostly that of the up and down motion of its center of gravity, especially when walking slowly. The direction of the motion is actually achieved by leaning forward (or backward or sideward). So the idea of rolling along on our feet makes no sense, we actually bob up and down whilst leaning in order to push our center of gravity forwards - and there's a natural, efficient way of doing it.

The forefoot should touch the ground first. You may also have come across the idea that the mid-foot touches the ground first, but because of the concave form of the foot, this is clearly impossible.

WELCOME TO THE JUNGLE

Another way of looking at natural walking and how it has evolved is going for a walk in the forest – barefoot. A few years ago I was hiking with friends through mountains and forest. At one point I abandoned my minimal shoes and went completely barefoot.

I realized at that point, that the whole idea of the heel-strike could only develop in a world with streets. When you walk on ever changing ground, which is never perfectly flat, you must touch with your forefoot first in order to keep your balance.

When you use the heel strike, your body weight is transferred to the foot as soon as you touch the ground. This is fine on a street if you wear shoes. In a forest where there are stones or thorns that could hurt your foot, this would be a very dangerous strategy. Touching with your forefoot first allows you to "scan" the ground for dangers before transferring your body weight. This allows you to feel whether it's safe to transfer your weight first. The other advantage is that as you collect information about the ground before you transfer your weight, the brain has time to work out how best to keep its balance.

The forefoot strike simply allows you to be much more in control and sure-footed.

So, if you are a fervent defender of the heel strike, take a walk in the jungle, a forest or up a mountain with your bare feet. You will find out just how useful and natural the forefoot strike is.

Plus, it's great fun!

ON WALKING AND RUNNING STYLES

Optimal human gait is defined by bio-mechanics, gravity and the ground we walk on. It is the same for all humans. It is therefore all the more astonishing that people develop such different running or walking styles. Just as we can recognize friends from far away by looking at their posture, some people also develop unique walking or running styles.

But then, how many different walking or running styles have you seen in cats or bears? The reason why it is so difficult to identify a cat at night is that their moving patterns are all almost identical, even if their personalities are not. This is because they all follow their natural movement patterns, defined by genetics and gravity hard-wired into their brains. The human brain comes with much less hard-wiring and can learn more unnatural movement. This is why we have ballet dancing or the moon walk, which is cool, but is of course unnatural movement that will often become painful when it becomes the default way of moving.

So even though we are not all made to a "norm" or look exactly the same, we should still obey the same anatomical and physical laws and have quite similar movement patterns. When someone walks with one or both feet pointing sideways, stiff knees or a pelvis that doesn't tilt from side to side (men should move their hips when they walk too!) this individual pattern is in fact nothing but the expression of a dysfunctional body. All these "deviations" can lead to pain and abnormal joint abrasion.

This should also lead you to question the point of "running analysis", or, specifically, the conclusions of running analysis. Some people have specialists look at their running style to help them choose the right running shoes. Indeed, many people have running styles so far from the original natural pattern that they cannot run without special gear that will supposedly alleviate the damage done to their joints.

This strikes me as being very much like mounting a sail on your broken car instead of repairing the motor. Is it really that clever to help a person who has lost the capacity to run, the way our species was designed to, to run even more?

Bad running style is mostly symptomatic of dysfunctional body parts. Any running style that differs from the simple natural running movement consists of extra compensatory movement. This comes at the cost of reduced efficiency and higher joint abrasion.

If you have an unusual or inefficient running or walking technique, I suggest you first see a good therapist who will help you understand and resolve the issues that make your running dysfunctional. What is the point of going running every day if you are doing it wrong? Would you jump head first against the wall every day to strengthen your leg muscles?

TLDR

Humans achieve walking by creating an up or downward movement in their hinge joints, i.e. their ankles, knees and pelvis. The energy of the downward movement is absorbed mainly in the connective tissue in the foot and the Achilles tendon. Like a tensed rubber band, this energy can then be converted into forward movement.

However, this shock absorbing and energy saving walk can only be achieved if and when the foot naturally touches the ground with the forefoot first. In the unnatural but common heel strike gait, the shock very audibly goes straight into the knee joint. The foot being concave, the often-proclaimed "roll off the heel" idea is nothing but a dangerous myth.

It is worth repeating: unnatural walking and running styles are a sign of a dysfunctional body. They should not be artificially compensated for with inlays or special running shoes. It is far more sensible to work on the underlying problems with a good therapist before training, otherwise you will simply be repeating harmful moving patterns that will create more damage.

3
IS SITTING THE NEW CANCER?

Sitting is the new cancer.

Tim Cook

How to alleviate the worst effects of our sedentary lifestyle with an active sitting posture. What most people misunderstand about sitting. Choosing the right office chair.

SITTING — HOW DANGEROUS IS IT REALLY?

"Sitting is the new cancer" says Apple CEO Tim Cook and presents a watch that will remind you to get up regularly and walk around a bit. Indeed, our sedentary lifestyle is unanimously considered to be one of the main reasons for the back-pain epidemic.

In fact, when you sum up the time spent eating, working, watching TV or using your computer, it might turn out that you spend more time sitting than sleeping. So it is not surprising that most people will sooner or later experience back problems after long periods of sitting.

It is therefore astonishing that there is virtually no information about healthy sitting to be found. We often hear that we should "get up every 30 minutes". This is indeed useful, but quite beside the point.

What is much more important, is that how you sit will make a big difference in the long run. What one sits on is of course also very important. With most chairs, you will simply never get a chance to sit correctly.

The good news is that if you do it right and chose the right chair, you can sit for hours without causing major problems. While sitting will never exactly be a healthy workout, it does not have to be as damaging as smoking. What you need, therefore, in sitting as in walking, standing and any other type of movement, is really good *movement quality*.

GENERAL OBSERVATIONS ON MOVEMENT QUALITY

How you do something is more important than what you do.

But what does quality of movement actually mean? Let's take the example of drinking a cup of coffee. When you lift the cup off the table and bring it towards your mouth, several things must happen.

The right muscles must perform the action

Once you have grabbed the cup, your deltoid muscles will also have to lift the elbow while your biceps will have to bend it in order to bring the cup closer to the mouth. The biceps will also turn the hand when you tilt the cup.

These are (some of) the muscles, which perform the actual desired action.

The antagonists of these muscles must stay relaxed

All muscles have antagonists, i.e. muscles performing the opposite movement. In our example, the triceps straightens the arm and the latissimus dorsi muscle pulls down the elbow if the arm is raised. Antagonists have to be completely relaxed, otherwise the muscles performing the desired action have to work harder - which is a waste of energy and makes coordination harder.

This might seem obvious, but for example in martial arts, beginners often use the biceps when they punch. Punching requires straightening your arm with the triceps, but beginners will often use the biceps when hitting the target because it makes them feel stronger.

The body must stay balanced and stable

But drinking a cup of coffee does not just happen thanks to your arm. Whether you stand or sit, as your arm extends towards the cup, your body has to keep its balance. Every tiny muscle in the body has to adapt to a movement and adjust for perfect balance at all times. For example, maybe your toes will have to push against the ground harder as your arm goes forward to avoid falling over.

No superfluous use of muscle

When drinking or writing people often pull their shoulders forward with their pectoralis muscles or hold them up with their trapezius muscle (Remember Figure 1.3!). Though these muscles are not antagonists working against the movement, they are not necessary to achieve the desired result of cup-to-mouth. Not only do such movements not appear aesthetic as natural movement does, but they also usually come at the cost of poorer balance.

All useful action-muscles should be used

Take a bottle of water from the kitchen counter and give it to your partner or friend. You can lift the bottle just with your biceps. Or else, you can slightly bend your knee when you grab the bottle and the use leg and arm to lift the bottle. The latter is more efficient and keeps the body moving as one.

Any movement should be supported by and performed with your whole body. Do not isolate muscle groups (see chapter on strength training).

The benefits of good movement quality

When you employ all the right muscles, your functional strength is much greater. You also have better coordination, stability and balance. Natural movement patterns create much less abrasion on the joints.

HOW TO SIT RIGHT

When people learn that I'm a body worker, a funny spasm often goes through their spine. They immediately try to stand or sit ultra-straight, thinking that this is considered good posture. It's not.

Your spine is not, as the German or French language would have it, a vertebral column, or a spinal column. A healthy spine takes the shape of a double S, which is definitely not one of the most popular shapes for columns.

Form follows function: Because spines and columns perform different functions, they have different shapes. Columns, for one, are usually designed to stand perfectly still. If your spine did the same you would not be able breathe. Natural breathing - the lifting of the rib cage with your scalene muscles and the up and down movement of your diaphragm - creates an undulation in your spine.

Exercise 1:

In a relaxed upright stance, breathe slowly and deeply. Keep your lower back and neck as relaxed as possible. As you slowly breathe in and out, feel the gentle wave-like movement going through the spine. Exaggerate your breathing movement so that you can really feel how your spine moves with it.

This spine movement creates subtle, constantly changing pressure on your discs, which stimulates them. It also keeps the erector muscles active at all times.

Now you understand that sitting, just like standing, is a movement, not a position. The only "position" you will ever be in is when you stop breathing, at which point I'm afraid you will be about to fall off you perch…

Exercise 2:

Sit on your hands, with the palms facing upwards and the back of your hands on the chair. The bones you feel in contact with your hands are called sitting bones (Figure 3.1). They are rounded and will let you place your center of gravity either slightly behind them or in front of them. The former will encourage your back to lean against the back of the chair and your pelvis will tilt backwards, your pubic bone will come up. This is called a retro-version of the pelvis, it will result in an ante-version, letting the torso go forwards and the pubic bone go down. You will in fact be sitting in between your sitting bones and your coccyx (Figure 3.2).

Also, watch one of my sitting exercises on YouTube[6].

If your torso's center of gravity is slightly in front of the sitting bone, you will sit on your sitting bones and your femur.

Try both solutions and evaluate how well each of them lets you breathe.

You will find that if your back rests against the back of the chair, breathing is difficult. In fact, the retroversion of the pelvis will pull you into a hunchback position, which in turn pushes your sternum down on your diaphragm. This will result in very shallow breathing and virtually no spine movement at all. The fact that part of your body weight now rests on your coccyx makes this sitting posture even more uncomfortable.

If you have paid extra-money for an "ergonomic" chair, this means that you have lumbar support. On the upside, your lower back will lose less of its lordosis (inward curvature of the spine) and the pelvis will be in a better position, but on the downside, this impedes spine movement even further, thus encouraging muscle and disc atrophy. As a general rule, as I mentioned in the chapter on shoes, every time you let a machine or an item of clothing, or in this case, furniture, do the job for you, your body will in time lose the capacity to do these things itself and the luxury or help will become a necessity that you depend on. This is true for soft shoes, inlays, lumbar support, sometimes even wheelchairs and glasses. They are tools that might be useful for a limited time; but is always good to avoid developing lazy legs, feet or eyes.

---

6   https://youtu.be/aspaDM2npcw

Many people think that sitting with your torso leaning forwards slightly requires tremendous muscle strength. It doesn't. The reason this posture is considered difficult is that most people overstretch their spine when they try this. They use their posas (bend the hip

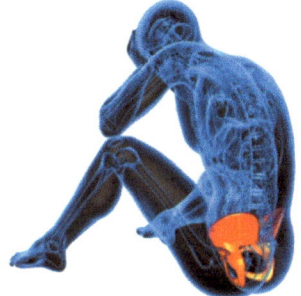

Figure 3.1

The pelvis makes contact with the ground through the sitting bones. Note their round shape. This will encourage you to either tilt your pelvis forwards or backwards - depending on the angle of your torso.

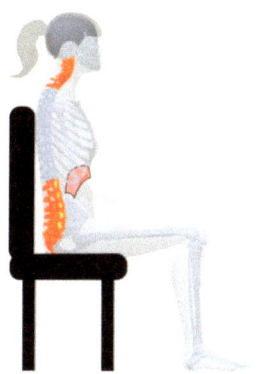

Figure 3.2

When the center of gravity of your torso is behind the sitting bone, the pelvis rolls backwards and you end up sitting between your sitting bones and your coccyx. This is not only very uncomfortable, but it also pushes the head forward. In this way, leaning backwards not only creates lower back pain, but also tension in the neck.

joint) and quadratus lumborum (QL) muscles, along with the erector muscles of the spine, to overextend their lower back in particular (Figure 3.3 – left).

This is unnecessary and harmful. There are many reasons for the QL being *the* back pain muscle. One of them is that this muscle if often permanently contracted (Figure 3.3 – right). This overuse will frequently result in decreased blood flow and some nerve types will then signal pain to encourage movement.

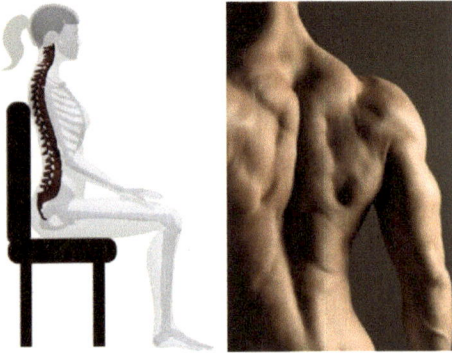

Figure 3.3

When people try to correct their sitting posture, they often push out their chest and try to sit up "straight". This puts even more pressure on the lower back, which becomes over-extended. It is also very hard work for the muscles involved. This is the reason why no one can actually maintain a "straight sitting posture" for more than a few minutes - which is just as well, because this particular posture is quite as harmful as the slouching sitting posture.

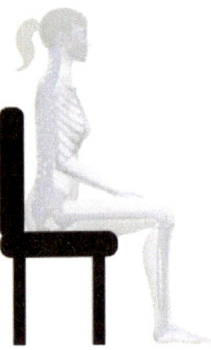

Figure 3.4

In order to have good sitting posture, the torso's center of gravity should be slightly in front of the sitting bone. You can then completely relax your lower back, especially the quadrates lumborum and the hip flexor (psoas-illiacus) muscle. Only then will your spine truly allow for a relaxed and relaxing breathing movement.

In fact, when the center of gravity of your torso is slightly in front of your sitting bones, you can relax your lower back completely. You will guiltily feel like a lazy sack of potatoes, but that state of complete relaxation will actually allow for the breathing movement to happen naturally. The resulting undulation is all you need to keep the back muscles in constant movement and to stimulate your discs (Figure 3.4).

Now switch your attention to your legs. To start, keep your knees at an angle slightly wider than 90 degrees. Your feet should be flat on the ground. When your torso goes forward, usually while you breathe out, your bodyweight will have to be partially transferred through your legs. Make sure this is the case; it will keep your leg muscles permanently active while you sit.

Not using one's legs is in fact one of the main reasons people never find a good sitting posture. Most people cross their ankles and pull back their feet under their chair. This makes their legs completely inactive and encourages a backward tilt of the pelvis. It makes it impossible not to slouch after a minute or two.

When you do use your legs, not only is it easier to have the pelvis remain in a slightly tilted forward position, but your leg muscles are actually activated, which is not only good for the muscles themselves. Activating your leg muscles also helps the blood and lymph circulate better. This will simply give you more energy to get through a long working day.

The correct sitting posture is relaxing and keeps your back in permanent movement.

Again, Do Not Overstretch Your Lower Back!!

Keep it completely relaxed.

In the beginning, this posture might still be a little tiring after a few hours. You are allowed to rest after you have made the effort, so don't hesitate to use the back of your chair or your lumbar support - when you need it and after making the (very slight) effort. In fact, it may well be that after a few weeks of sitting correctly you will able to sit through a whole working day without needing any support and you will get up with a nicely relaxed back.

CHAIRS FROM HELL

The road to hell is paved with good intentions. Unfortunately, people who design chairs fall victim to the same traps as running shoe designers.

They want to "support the spine" or "allow the back to fully relax". The problem with ergonomic chairs, with lumbar support and arm-rests, is that they are so good at making you comfortable that your muscles have virtually no work at all to do. This can be a good thing, when they are tired, but it's a bad thing when they never have to work out at all.

A chair like this will act like a cast - it will certainly stabilize your body, but make your muscles weaker every day. As your muscles get weaker day by day, you will eventually actually need a chair with lumbar support, the way you would end up needing a wheelchair if you really were no longer able to use your legs.

So, what makes a good chair?

First of all, just like your feet need a firm ground to stand on, your sitting bones need a firm and stable surface to sit on. Very soft cushions on chairs or sofas do not offer the necessary resistance that your pelvis and spine need to stabilize against gravity through proper alignment. Again, imagine a skyscraper built on a swamp.

For this reason, sitting on big inflatable balls does not result in good sitting posture and is not even a good workout. It can only achieve tense muscles.

This surface has to be horizontal or very slightly angled to encourage an ante-version (forward position) of the pelvis. You can sometimes find a reversed angle in lounging chairs or in airports. These chairs will encourage you to lean back and are good only for relaxing and sleeping, but never for working, as they make sitting up and

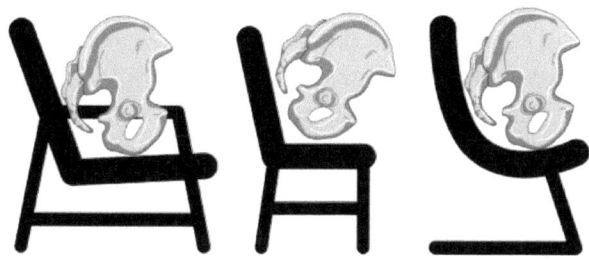

Figure 3.5

Chairs with round or backwards-sloping seats will encourage your pelvis to roll backwards (chair on the left and right). This will cause you to put a part of your body weight on your coccyx and will result in slouching. Only flat or very slightly angled forwards seats allow your pelvis to rest in an ante-version (forward) posture, which is a conditio-sine-qua-non for a relaxed and up-right sitting posture (chair in the middle).

looking in front of you very difficult (Figure 3.5).

As The Guardian newspaper reports[7] , even such simple anatomical facts are sadly ignored by European Standards, which allow chairs to slope backwards by 5 degrees. This is madness and starts a

---

7   http://www.theguardian.com/lifeandstyle/shortcuts/2015/apr/19/children-bad-backs-un-comfortable-school-chairs-campaign

vicious circle for all school children forced to sit in these chairs for hours every day.

Make sure your chair has the right height, too. Your sitting bones have to be slightly higher than your knees in order to allow the body weight to be supported by your legs. If the chair is too low and your knees too high, they will push the pelvis backwards and your spine into a slouching position.

Some office chairs come with wheels. Should you ever Google *sitting posture* you will find lots of pictures on the right sitting posture with people sitting on office chairs with wheels.

These pictures usually make at least two fundamental errors: A person sitting correctly with natural spine movement has to slightly push his or her feet into the ground when the body moves forward. This pressure in the legs will make the chair roll backwards.

The second error is that the person often sits too far back in the chair, which also makes using the legs difficult (Figure 3.6).

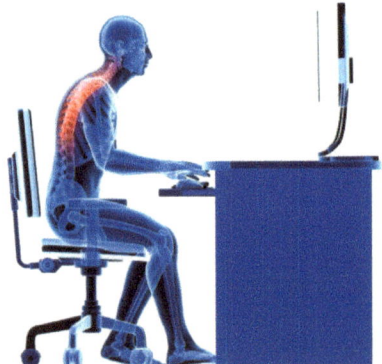

Figure 3.6
Office chairs with wheels do not allow for good posture. As you lean slightly forward, your chair can roll backwards. This is why most people pull their legs under the chair, which results in the bad sitting posture shown above.

TLDR

A typical, but very harmful sitting posture consists of leaning against the back of the chair, the knees bent and the feet under the chair. This position impedes a natural breathing movement in the spine and makes your legs useless. This position also relies on sitting on the coccyx instead of the sitting bones and hamstrings.

With the center of gravity of the torso in front of the sitting bones and the feet firmly on the ground, quite the opposite happens. The spine will be constantly moving with the breathing movement and the erector muscles will keep it up, while the muscles in the legs will transfer part of the body weight while you lean slightly forwards. This is called an active sitting posture.

A common mistake consists of trying to sit straight, which goes against the natural form of the spine and will result in its overextension. The muscles involved in this overextension will soon grow tired and start aching.

4
A STRONG BACK
KNOWS NO PAIN - OR DOES IT?

Why big muscles do not prevent back pain. Why exercise often actually makes you weaker. What is the goal of exercise or working out? Why animals do not have to work out, but you should.

MYTHS ABOUT STRONG BACKS

If you have started creating a healthier environment by choosing a better chair and wearing minimalist shoes, you may start thinking about working out or strengthening your muscles. When a person is slouching it looks like he or she does not have the strength to resist gravity. Surely with a bit more strength, one could "pull oneself together" and assume a nice upright, Prussian posture?

In order to achieve such a magnificent military posture and fight back pain, physiotherapy and strength training may seem like a good idea. The idea that "a strong back knows no pain" and that we need to tone our muscles, is a die-hard myth. Unfortunately, this misconception is being kept alive by many doctors, coaches, osteopaths and physiotherapists, who still happily prescribe strength training out of sheer habit and against all logical reason.

How dare I? Well, first of all, the number of strong backs which experience severe back pain is in fact quite high and has actually put an end to many a promising career. Such was the case for former Ukrainian boxing heavy weight champion Vladimir Klitschko, who had a slipped disk.

Tiger Woods has also had to abandon tournaments due to severe back pain and according to the Daily Telegraph, Usain Bolt suffers from such bad back problems that he can only sleep in a specially designed bed.

Body builders and weightlifters exchange tips and advice on where to get the best back operation every day in Internet forums.

This evidence should be enough to at least get health professionals thinking.

The truth is that good posture and natural movement are a result of relaxation and using the body in the right way. You can test this in a very simple way:

Exercise:

Stand up and feel what posture you are in. Try and have the best possible posture. You will know that your posture is good when you feel lighter, stronger and better balanced at the same time.

Which muscles do you have to tense to achieve this? Is there a single muscle in your body that would have to be stronger in order for you to achieve good posture?

There isn't. You probably realize that bad posture is a result of unnecessary tension in some body parts and not of weak muscles. This is true, whether you're sitting, standing, walking, dancing or cooking a meal.

Just think of children. They get to have good posture without having to be miniature versions of Arnold Schwarzenegger[8]. They are also

---

8   Nowadays, body-builders often have comprehensive knowledge about nutrition and

often surprisingly strong. This is because functional strength does not come from big muscles, but from a clever, uninhibited brain.

Therefore, if you want good posture, you need to learn to relax your muscles.

WHY STRENGTH TRAINING CREATES MORE PROBLEMS THAN IT SOLVES

When people do physiotherapy they often do experience an improvement in their physical condition and less back pain. This is only to be expected if they had an activity deficit in their daily routines before. It is not so much the gain in strength that will help them, but simply the increase in physical activity.

Still, strength training often creates more problems than it solves in the long run. This is because back pain often results from an excess of tone, a condition that gets even worse with conventional strength training.

The first myth that needs debunking is the idea that you need to strengthen your stomach muscles, most of all the rectus abdominis, commonly known as the "six-pack". Certain people who have not paid attention in Anatomy 101, but claim medical proficiency, will insist that these muscles support the weight of the torso.

What they fail to understand is the simple fact that your six pack is a muscle designed to lift up your pubic bone, pull down your sternum, or both, and therefore enable you to round your back. It is a flexor muscle that bends your pelvis-thigh joint, just like the

anatomy and are much more intelligent and informed than the cliché suggests. Please don't mistake my comments on strength training or bodybuilding for "workout bashing" because one can do much worse than undertake regular serious workouts.

biceps bends your arm. A really strong biceps will bend your arm even better but it will not become a tensor and straighten your arm.

In the same way, a stronger six-pack will be able to bend your back even better, but will never, ever help you straighten it.

One can only marvel at how such an obvious anatomic contradiction is still being mindlessly repeated over and over again, but you will see that there are a few more obvious fallacies in fitness-related issues that will be dealt with here.

Back to our strong stomach muscles: Not only can they not help you straighten up from your hunchback posture, they will actually encourage such a position. There is a mechanical, a psychological and a neurologic reason for this.

Mechanically, when you do strength training and a muscle gets bigger, it is actually the diameter that increases. The origin and insertion of a muscle cannot change; therefore the increase in volume can only affect the diameter. This changes the natural relation between length and width of the muscle. Every muscle has a natural tension and this tension will only increase as the muscle becomes bigger. The basic force with which your rectus abdominis pulls down your rib cage will therefore go up.

Now some clever person might say: "No problem, I'll make my back muscles stronger, too". This would ignore the fact that the overall tension on the spine will increase. Imagine a circus tent that stands with the "right" tension. Now if someone tries to make it "stronger" or make it stand up even better by pulling all the strings and ropes even tighter, the overall tension goes up, the tent becomes stiffer and there is more tension on the poles which will have a tendency to bend and deform.

The same is true for the spine. If you look closely at its anatomy, you will see that while you have muscles that can turn and bend the spine, you really don't have any to extend or straighten it. Good posture depends on lowering tension, not adding to it.

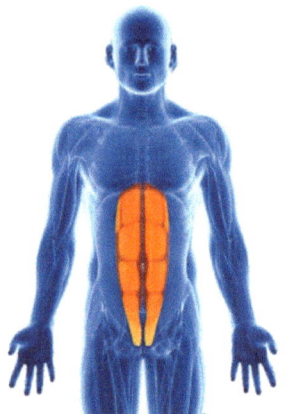

Figure 4.1

The rectus abdominis muscle can pull the rib cage down or lift up the pubic bone or both. It is a flexor muscle that achieves a round back.

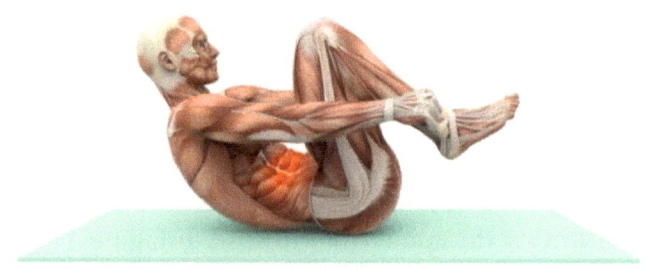

Figure 4.2

This is a typical exercise to strengthen the rectus abdominis muscle. However well you train this muscle, it will always be a flexor for the spine. When over-trained, it will constantly pull your rib cage down and thus encourage slouching.

Too much tension results in bad posture, but bad posture will then in turn create even more tension. For example, if your stomach muscles are too tight, they will pull the torso down and bring the head forward. Thus the neck will have to work harder and tension will go up. Also, the back will become rounder. Because of the effect of leverage, the lower back muscles, the quadratus lumborum muscles, now have more work to do to stabilize the torso.

These muscles already have to provide an unnatural amount of work at all times, they surely do not need to be trained even more. Their muscle tone is much too high as it is. They need to relax and move, not to work more and hold.

Even if someone did have a muscle that was too weak, would it be intelligent to then go to a club or a physiotherapist and train that muscle?

No, it wouldn't. Because if someone does not have the necessary strength in one muscle to function well in everyday life, that raises the question of why it is not being used sufficiently. So instead of having to train that muscle twice a week, it would seem more useful to teach the person how to use it sufficiently in everyday life.

So, is there no such thing as "a lack of muscle tone"? Well, yes there is. Ironically, this is usually the result of exaggerated muscle tone in the antagonists. A well-trained therapist will correctly identify these situations. A very well-trained therapist, instead of telling you to train this muscle you never use, will relax the antagonist and correct your posture in such a way, that from then on you will be using that muscle.

Life is not about training, it's about living. No animal picks up weights and trains. Not even man's best friend, however well trained. They do use their bodies correctly though and as long as they get the right quantity of movement, the quality of their everyday movements is sufficient to keep them in good shape and avoid back pain. Take a leaf out of their book. It obviously works.

You shouldn't have to waste your time with pointless strengthening and stretching (see next chapter) exercises. You should live an active life and move well.

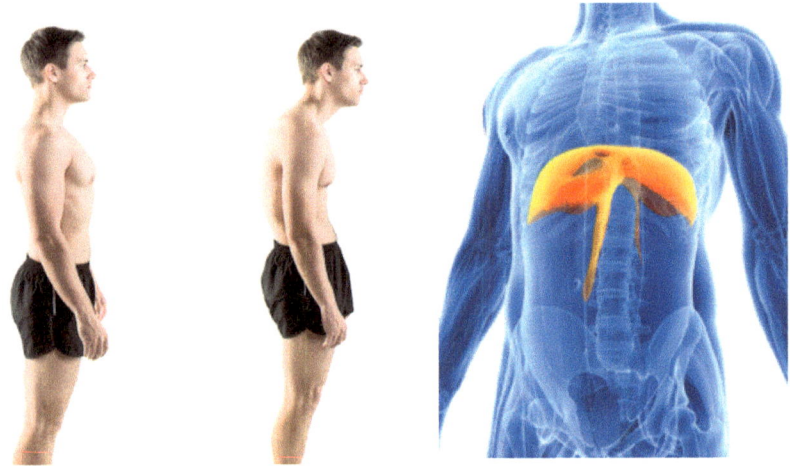

Figure 4.3

The origin of the rectus abdominis is right behind your sternum. Only a long and relaxed muscle allows the rib cage to go up sufficiently in order to breathe deeply (left). People often put extra tension on this muscle because they think it makes them look thinner or more muscular. The body structure on the right hand side seems exaggerated, but body-workers encounter it quite often. Observe the position of the diaphragm. It becomes obvious that deep and relaxed breathing is impossible when the rectus abdominis muscle is too tense.

THE FLAT STOMACH HABIT

The other reason why you shouldn't train your six-pack is psychological. Magazines are full of pictures of people with dysfunctional rectus abdominis muscle and low body fat who tighten

76

these muscles when the picture is taken. The result is that ordinary people think this is a desirable and attractive standard that they should strive to achieve.

As I have pointed out previously, your rib cage has to rise in order to allow you to breathe in easily and ventilate your lungs. If the muscle tone in your six-pack is too high, it will permanently drag your rib cage down and allow for superficial breathing only.

People enjoy the feeling of a flat stomach and assume it makes them attractive. They will therefore try to constantly keep the stomach muscle under tension. This will make their breathing even shallower and round the back even more.

It is particularly ironic that this posture, with the tummy pulled in and the pelvis tilted backwards is considered so attractive when in fact, this particular angle of pelvis is a common cause for a dysfunctional pelvic floor. This, in turn, often results in a lowered sex drive and less fulfilling physical relations.

Last but not least, there are neurological implications to training the stomach. People who do strength training and obsess over their six-pack like to use it as often as possible. The idea that they look better and need more training leads them to over-use their rectus abdominis even in training situations where this is unnecessary.

But neurons that fire together wire together. That is to say that moving patterns are created where the six-pack is uselessly tensed when this is actually counterproductive.

This can easily be observed when people tie their shoes. Instead of just relaxing and bending their knees, people first hold their breath (always a sign of bad quality of movement), tighten their front and make a round back and only when they can not bend further down do they bend the knees.

This is both inefficient and not very graceful and typical in people who use their spine-flexor muscle when they shouldn't.

HOW STRENGTH TRAINING CREATES INEFFICIENT MOVEMENT PATTERNS

And it was quite interesting to see where my swing was then and how much force I could generate with a very skinny frame. How did I do that? How do I generate that much power? That's kind of what we are getting back into.

Tiger Woods (2014)

This is also the reason why most strength training actually makes you weaker. Because while the individual, isolated muscle does of course become stronger with training, many, in fact almost all exercises create bad moving patterns, which reduce your functional strength.

Push-ups are a good example of this, even if they have the virtue of training much more than one isolated muscle. Push-ups are in fact a very efficient method for training upper body strength and as these exercises go, much better than the butterfly machine used in strength training which really only trains your pectoralis muscle.

But there is still a catch that makes you lose functional strength. This is because the "right" way to do this exercise is to keep your body as stiff as an ironing board while your arms push it off the ground. Again, neurons that fire together wire together, therefore you train your body to respect a pattern by which the hips are kept stiff when the arms exert forward power.

Mentally turn the push-up exercise by ninety degrees. Observe a person pushing a heavy door. Most people will now tighten their stomach, pull the pelvis forward and open the door with a round back. Or, just as bad, hold the body as straight and still as they do when doing push-ups. Again, you can tell by the fact that they also have to hold their breath while pushing the door open.

The efficient and natural way to open a door lets the pelvis tilt forwards a bit and glide backwards before starting to push. This is what you do naturally when it gets really difficult, for example when you push a car. The same thing should happen, though not as visibly, when you open a door. Not only will you have better balance, your arms will also be helped by other muscles in your body and the door won't feel quite as heavy.

Again, these slight differences may not matter when you are twenty. But they will make a difference when you are seventy or older. Changing these patterns will become more and more difficult with age because they become hard-wired. Better to start doing it right today.

In a way, most exercises in strength training create artificial problems that shouldn't occur in real life (pushing up your body only with your arms for example). Because these are harder to do, you must then train, so you have the strength to actually perform these inefficient movements.

However, for those who enjoy solving problems they created in the first place, strength training is only second best. Stretching is an even worse waste of time - unless you copy your children or your cat, that is.

TLDR

Strength training is an allocated time period in a week during which a person tries to compensate for bad posture and inefficient movement patterns by isolating inactive muscles and giving them a good workout.

This approach usually produces satisfying short-term pain relief, especially when the pain was caused by a lack of activity. It does not, however, resolve the actual issue and will stop working as soon as the person stops working out.

A movement is only natural, efficient and healthy when the body acts as one. Almost all strengthening exercises rely on keeping parts of the body stiff. Therefore, while some inactive muscles get a nice workout, even more inefficient movement patterns are learned.

Therefore, the more the person trains, the more he or she learns to be inefficient in every day life. He or she will have to work out even more to counteract this. It is the beginning of a vicious circle

which is also very time consuming.

5
STRETCHING – A DANGEROUS WASTE OF TIME

Pain is the best teacher.

Unattributed

Why there can be no such thing as a "shortened muscle". Why you touching your toes with a straight knee will never stretch your hamstrings. Why stretching creates harmful and useless moving patterns. Why you can just forget about stretching altogether.

SHORT MUSCLES?

Many people will tell you that they have "short muscles". They are often deluded into thinking that a muscle will become shorter with age or lack of use and can be made longer again by stretching. This is, again, a misconception that is mindlessly repeated in the media and by people selling stretching classes.

The muscles, or rather the group of muscles that people will insist on telling you is too short, are the hamstrings. This group of mainly three muscles (semitendinosus, semimembranosus, biceps femoris long & short head) is situated at the back of your thigh and can bend the knee and straighten the hip. They originate in your sitting bone (ischial tuberosity) and insert in your lower leg, the tibia and fibula.

Now, some people make other people try to touch their feet with their hands without bending their knees. Supposedly, if you can't do this, or if this hurts too much, you have "short hamstrings".

Let's ask some simple questions - for example, what exactly is a short(ened) muscle? As you know, muscles have origins and insertions. These are simply anatomical terms for saying both ends. For our hamstrings that would roughly be the sitting bones on one end and the tibia and fibula (lower leg bones) on the other end (see Figure 5.1).

Now, when someone talks about short hamstrings, does that mean that those two ends, where the muscle attaches through tendons to the bones, have now moved closer together? Do my hamstrings not go as far as my lower leg anymore, but attach to a point above the knee? Of course not.

Here is another question that mystifies doctors, yoga teachers and physiotherapists:

If I want to stretch, say, a rubber band, I will grab it at both ends and pull them further and further apart. In order to stretch a muscle, the insertion and the origin would have to move further away from one another too.

Now put a straight leg on a chair and slowly bend forward to grab your foot. Pay attention to your knee and sitting bone. It will turn out that they barely move at all.

Try again with the other all time classic: from a standing position with straight knees, bend forwards and touch your toes with your hands. Again, funnily, the two ends of the hamstrings hardly moved.

So where does the pain come from, since the muscle is obviously hardly being stretched at all?

Thousands of older people get diagnosed every year with

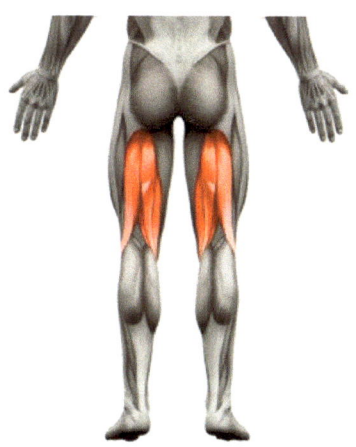

Figure 5.1
Your hamstring muscles.

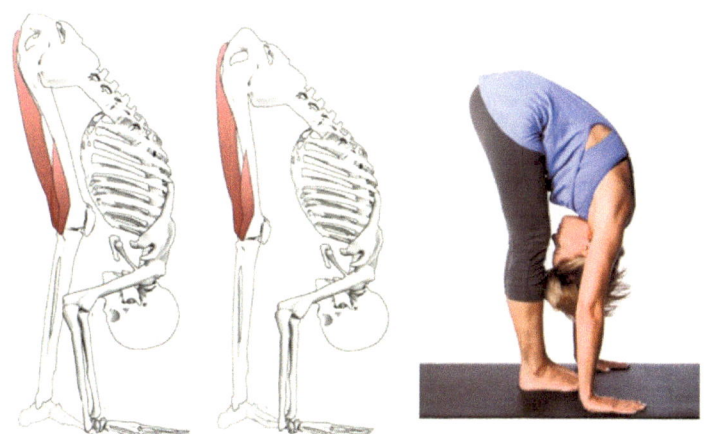

Figure 5.2
This is a useless exercise. First of all, the distance between the sitting bones and the insertion of the muscles does not change as you bend forward, so an actual stretching effect is questionable at best. Worse, it creates inefficient movement patterns. You have knees so that you can bend them when you need to, for example, to pick up something from the floor. Many people do not bend their knees enough in everyday life as it is. Why would anyone train to keep the knees even stiffer?

"contracted capsules" or "shortened muscles", for example before they have a hip replacement. Funnily enough, these restrictions of mobility often completely disappear under general anesthetic. In fact, most of us could do perfect splits in these conditions.

Again, where are the short muscles?

Well, the good news is, you don't have any. You do not have to stretch your muscles because they do not really get shorter.

Moreover, we are yet to see a single study that finds any actual benefits in stretching. In fact, most studies come to the conclusion that stretching is mostly useless at best and potentially harmful in the worst cases. Do not stretch!

Or rather, stretch like your cat or your children. The way you do when you get out of bed, just longer. Real stretching is a pleasure.

The difference, and this is where we learn why your hamstrings hurt when they don't get stretched, is that your typical stretching class movements go against all principles of biomechanics, while your morning stretches are actually natural and useful.

The pain caused in the hamstring-stretching example is not due to a muscle being stretched. It isn't, as a clever person might suspect, the myofascial link from these muscles to other body parts, though this does play a role. It is in fact your nervous system, crying out: "Use your knees, dude!" It is really that simple! Our nervous system is there to protect us from harm and sends the pain signal early enough to prevent us from really hurting ourselves.

We have knees so we can use them. The knee joint is there to bring the pelvis and the ankles closer together. If you refuse to use it, how can you be astonished that it's a) difficult to reach your feet, and b) painful?

All you do here is create an artificial problem (touch your toes without bending the knees) and then train to solve it. This is very much like trying to win a car race using only first gear.

Why would anyone refrain, under pain, from using one joint and then come to the conclusion that they need to make a different body part more flexible? Who told people to do this?

If you want to look behind you, you turn your neck, your torso and your pelvis. If you chose to only use your neck, you can't turn 180°. Does that mean you have to stretch your neck muscles? No, it means you need to use your whole body.

If you try to join your hands behind your back without bending the elbows, do you then need to stretch your pectoralis muslces? Do you heck!

These are silly problems and there is no point in trying to find really clever solutions for them!

HOW LONG WOULD YOU LIKE IT?

Now for another embarrassing question… How long is it and how long would you like it? When somebody tells you to stretch a muscle, please ask them how they evaluated the current length of the muscle. What allows them to ascertain that it's too short?

As you already know, there really is no such thing as a shortened muscle, but there is such a thing as tension in the connective tissue around it and the flexibility of said tissue.

As a body worker I know that a runner needs rather tight hamstrings and has a pretty sturdy Achilles tendon. This provides better running efficiency, as the tissue will be able to store the "bouncing energy" better.

This tension that is useful for a runner is death to a ballet dancer though, as he or she needs to be able to lift the leg quite high.

In fact, in both cases the tissue has adapted its tension and resistance exactly to how it is used every day.

The next question to ask your fitness coach is therefore: How long would you like my muscles to be - or much more accurately: How flexible do I need my connective tissue to be?

You can see that only you can answer this. But you don't have to. Your connective tissue adapts to the use you make of it. You don't have to actively take control over this or be in charge. It happens automatically.

All you have to do is make the movements you wish to be able to do often enough and do them right. The tissue will follow and you will never have "short muscles".

SPORTS

Who told people they have be able to bench-press 200 kg and have biceps the size of a watermelon? Why do 11 millionaires have to run about after a single ball on a football field? Who came up with the idea that we have to run 42 km? The first guy who did this famously died yet we have a whole industry that tries to get us to do the same thing. Where is the use in spending a lifetime training so you can do the 100 meters in under one second? Is there any real life application to this?

Sports, in fact, mostly consist of artificially created problems. They can also be fun and make sure we get off the couch. Very commendable.

Sports are not, however, designed to give you better health. They are, in this respect, completely beside the point.

The reason that adults have to keep doing exercises to stay in good health is because what they do in everyday life is not good enough to keep them in good shape. Sports mostly try to make up in movement quantity what we lack in movement quality. Which doesn't work.

Something else sport cannot do is make up for a poor diet. The flat belly that is so desirable comes from the kitchen much more than the track.

Yes, the human species does need a minimum amount of physical activity and this is where sports have a role to play. But we would be much more successful in being healthy if what we do all day long was done well.

This is after all, what animals do. They learn movement through imitation and play as they grow. Once they are adults however, they just get on with the business of living. A cat has yet to be seen doing squats so it can jump further, or doing 45 minutes of stretching exercises.

Life is not about training, it's about living.

TRAIN THE BRAIN

But what should one train in order to keep fit? If strength training is mostly useless and stretching actually completely pointless, what should we train.

We should train the main organ that is responsible for our posture and our movement quality: The brain.

Unfortunately, most advice about posture and back pain comes from people in the fitness industry. They are obsessed with speed, distance, weight and measure success or progress accordingly.

They forget that voluntary movements (picking up a cup of coffee) as well as automatic movements (keeping the body in balance) are created in the brain and that the measure of success is quality, not quantity.

Did you do specific stretching or strengthening exercises to learn how to ride a bike? Or to learn how to throw a ball? These activities are 99% brain and 1% muscle and so is posture and everyday movement.

This is why stretching and strengthening exercises are 99% useless when it comes to learning posture and movement.

TRUE MASTERY - WHAT PHYSICAL ACTIVITY MAKES SENSE?

Humans do not have the strength of a bear. They do not have the flexibility of a snake or the speed of a cheetah. Some Kung-Fu styles famously take inspiration from other animals and their adepts try to learn from them.

But because humans are humans with human anatomy, this is ridiculous. Humans are good at one thing though, and that is being human and moving like humans.

At a certain point in our evolution the bipedal walk freed our hands, which in turn allowed us to use tools, which in turn allowed us to hunt and get more protein. These factors allowed us to grow the most powerful brain of all animals, which in turn allows us to play a Bach Sonata, dance a beautiful tango or juggle with flaming torches.

Most people stay short of their potential and only ever learn how to use their body well enough to get by in everyday life, although some humans do take pleasure in mastery.

An engineer will learn how to play the guitar although it is not absolutely necessary for getting by in everyday life, it's just for the pleasure of mastery. Likewise, a doctor might learn to paint beautiful pictures.

Humans can learn to play golf or tennis and enjoy mastering a technique or a game. But this is mastery of a specific skill set rather than mastery of everyday physical movement.

Some readers may be familiar with the 1970 classic Jonathan Livingston Seagull by Richard Bach about a seagull who takes pleasure in improving its flying skills beyond what is necessary for a seagull to survive.

His fellow seagulls see this as a pointless activity but Jonathan persists and becomes good at flying, which is what a seagull does.

Humans, though not the fastest runners, most flexible contortionists or strongest animals do stand out in one respect: They are probably the most versatile species of the animal kingdom.

It is this flexibility, not of limb but of brain, that makes us human. And it is what keeps us healthy. It should not be something we train for an hour or two every day, only to then put "our bodies back in the cupboard". We should move like humans all day long - as efficiently and with as much grace as possible.

This does not mean dancing ballet. It means relaxing your shoulder when you lift a cup of coffee. It means letting your pelvis accompany your arm movement when you open a door. It means bending your knee when you open a drawer.

In short, humans should strive for mastery of the human way of moving. It is fulfilling and healthy.

A good activity therefore is one where you have time to concentrate on yourself, rather than on a ball and a goal. It is one that can be done very slowly, to give you time to feel what is happening. It is one where every movement happens in the whole body.

CLEVER PHYSICAL ACTIVITIES

Yoga is one of those clever disciplines, even though there are a great number of exercises, especially stretching exercises, which go against human biomechanics. Many yoga exercises are in fact not relevant in everyday life. Yoga does, however, often lead to a nicely honed and well-balanced body and is therefore still one of the more clever choices. Yoga comes in many different forms and styles. I suggest you choose a gentle and slow method. If your yoga teacher is also a body worker, this will guarantee you a deeper understanding of how yoga works and what it can achieve.

Another option is Latin dancing, such as salsa. Unlike the artificial ballet, salsa is all about relaxation and flexible strength. When I say salsa, please forget the artistic overdone version of salsa that is often shown on TV or YouTube channels. This is just gymnastics with music.

I mean the smooth, elegant salsa that seventy-year-olds dance in Cuba that is so much more appealing.

Personally I favor the style of martial arts, Senmotic red, which was developed from the Chinese WingChun fighting style. Senmotic red evolved with contemporary knowledge of physics and biomechanics into a style that is less harmful to your body and that of your opponent.

It has an immediate feedback system (you get hit) when you make an inefficient movement, which greatly accelerates the learning pace. The system was conceived and is taught in a way that emphasizes functionality. Because our body is always the same regardless of what we're doing, what is true in fighting is true in every day life and vice versa.

Without any extra training at all, Senmotic red practitioners often become extremely strong and fit. This does not come from endurance training, but from efficient use of the body.

TLDR

Humans should move like humans. Not like the humans you see in the street, but the way humans are designed to move.

We all do this pretty well when we are children, but then we copy our parents and teachers and go to school, where we are taught so sit passive and still on an un-ergonomic chair for hours at a time.

We learn this lesson well, which is why governments all over the world later have to pay for advertisements to encourage adults to do the opposite and move more.

By this time, we have made our bodies and brains stiff and have lost the capacity to move naturally. This is when we are told we need to stretch or exercise. What we really need to do is remember how we moved as kids and train our brain more than our muscles.

A well-trained brain will allow you to have good posture and keep active, even through long unhappy hours sitting at your office desk. Indeed, as the quantity of everyday movement and activity decreases with age, the quality at least should go up.

When writing, publishing and editing a book for example, you spend weeks and months in front of a computer. Fortunately, since I have read my book, my back wasn't passively leaning against the back of the chair. It was being used to stabilize my torso.

My spine was constantly moving slightly with my breathing and my legs were actively supporting my body weight. I worked on this book for about three months, sitting many hours a day. Practicing what I preach enabled me to avoid any discomfort.

Thank you, brain.

6
THE PSYCHOLOGY
OF BACK PAIN

*On the day that you feel that first twinge of back pain, an entire personal
history has already unfolded.*

Deepak Chopra

What embodiment is, what it proves and where Amy Cuddy went
wrong.

ON EMBODIMENT

How can you tell that someone is having a lousy day? By their
posture of course. Body language is a very accurate mood indicator
and we cannot help but notice or read someone's body language
at all times.

So, your mood influences your posture. When you are down (!),
you slouch and drag your feet. Being in love on a sunny day looks
quite different.

This isn't exactly exciting news. It does raise an interesting question
though: Does this also work the other way round? Can bad
slouching posture affect your mood?

It would appear so, as therapists know when they change someone's
posture by improving their body structure. Both my own personal
experience and feedback from patients confirms this. Around
the fifth session of fascia therapy, which focuses on the stomach,

supposedly the "emotional center" of the body, people often start thinking about or pursuing important life changes.

They get out of toxic relationships, start a new career or chose a healthier diet and lose weight. Making real life changes takes energy and a lot of self-confidence. These things often turn out to be at least as rewarding as the back pain relief itself for both the client and the therapist.

Until recently, this was a personal, anecdotal opinion.

This is why I'm very grateful to Amy Cuddy, social psychologist and professor and the Harvard Business School for having conducted an actual study on the influence of posture on self-confidence and stress management.

Her famous TED speech about the experiment is now the second most viewed TED speech ever, just behind the one on education by Sir Ken Robinson.

The experiment simply put one group of people in closed, hunched positions and the other group in open positions that take up a lot of space. She calls these the "open posture power poses".

Not surprisingly, at least for those with experience in the subject, it turns out that your posture has a major influence on your level of confidence and stress and your willingness to take risks.

When compared to their initial state, the power posers showed higher levels of testosterone (which indicates dominance) and lower levels of cortisol (which indicates stress), whereas it was exactly the other way round for the low power posers. A gambling test revealed that of course the power posers were more willing to take risks.

So, yes, you do not only slouch because you are sad or lack confidence, you also lack confidence because you slouch.

Amy Cuddy's excellent speech, which you really should watch[9] , did a lot to get people interested in the role posture plays in their life and career and in empowering women in particular.

But even though I'm very grateful that she raised so much awareness for the topic, I do believe she overlooks a very important point. First of all, her recommendation to assume a power pose for five minutes before a job interview implies that you do not have an open and confident posture by default. This is indeed true for most, but not all people.

A slouching, low-confidence posture has what we call an internal rotation. That means that the body in rolled in, the back is rounded, the head faces downward and the shoulders are hunched forwards. You might call this the hedgehog, bath tub or victim posture. Or simply an introverted posture.

Other people, often teachers or salespeople, have an extroverted posture. They pull back their shoulders and stick out their chest.

None of these postures are good or bad as such. They do make life difficult though when posture becomes structure, that means if the posture becomes the default state. This might seem like a good idea for the external rotated "confidence" structure. But while someone who knows how to stick out his or her chest will have less difficulty sticking up for themselves and getting their fair share of

9   http://www.ted.com/talks/amy_cuddy_your_body_language_shapes_who_you_ are?language=en

the pie, they might find it hard to be a good listener, encourage confidence in others, invite criticism and spend time alone.

Their posture might intimidate people and will make it harder for others to confide in you.

If your posture physically "gives space" to your interlocutor to express him or herself, he or she will find it easier to do so. While one posture gives you energy and confidence, another one might relax and calm you.

You need different postures for different life situations. Amy Cuddy assumes that people only ever have one posture and therefore one state of mind. While this is indeed true for most adults, it is not inevitable. Your body should remain flexible enough to stick your chest out for that important board meeting you have later today and then to deflate a bit when playing with your children or listening to your partner tell you about their day.

Never get stuck in one default posture. To be yourself, you have to have different sides. You have to be a dominant person in order to earn what you need and provide for yourself or family, but you also have to be a loving listening partner who can choose (!) to put themself second.

Only a flexible posture will make for a flexible and authentic person.

TLDR

Your posture changes depending on how you feel and how you feel depends partly on your posture and body structure. Changing one is changing the other. An authentic person has flexible posture and is a flexible being. He or she chooses how to react to a situation.

7
FINAL THOUGHTS

You experience the world you live in through your body. If your body has high muscle tension you will feel stressed. If you have a hunchback your posture tells a story of submission and you will have a hard time getting your share of the pie or that promotion that you want, simply because you constantly communicate that you are a victim. Victims aren't leaders.

You cannot separate mind and body - try leaving one at home and taking the other on a trip. Therefore, you do not just have a body, you are one.

If you have insurance for your car and your house, you get a new one if the car gets stolen or your house burns down. But health insurance? You can never insure your health, because no one can give it back to you when it's gone.

And because you only get one body, as you only get one you, you need to think about how much you value yourself.

How important is it to wear high heels to look good, if you sacrifice beautiful feet and good balance?

Is your back worth investing in a new mattress or minimal shoes, or is this too much of an investment and you'd rather get a fancier car or a nicer holiday.

How long would you like to be fit enough to play with your grandchildren? Do you still want to be able to dance at weddings when you're ninety years old?

It is sometimes fascinating to see how intelligent people have the most elaborate retirement plans. Financial retirement plans that is. People start planning their retirement in their forties. However, when you ask them what the most important thing is for older people, most will tell you that it is all about health. But if you ask about their strategy or what they invest today to still be alive and kicking tomorrow, they often don't have a clue or make any investments at all.

What kinds of problems run in the family? What kinds of illnesses does my lifestyle engender? What is it I want to be able to do till the day I die?

Health is not 100% predictable, but if you sit ten hours a day, or drink a bottle of wine every night or if your family seems genetically disposed to develop certain problems, it might be worth thinking about the possible consequences and what you can do to minimize the risks.

Because genetics is a capital you start with, you can't do much about it. You can however try to make the best of the cards you were dealt and start doing today what will make life worth living tomorrow. Or be a happy vegetable. That is, at least partly, your choice.

AUTHOR'S BIO

Peter Scholten, born in Germany in 1974 is an accomplished therapist and martial artist.

He started training at a young age in Judo, Taekwon-do and Jiu-Jitsu and then en- countered Bruce Lees Wing Chun (Wing Tsun) ghting style in the early 1990's. He opened his rst school in 1996 in Germany.

After fteen years of intensive training with some of the most renowned wing-chun practitioners, he met his current instructor, Frank W. Demann, in 2004, and immediately started learning Senmotic red, a very significant evolution from his former style.

Peter completed training as a fascia therapist in 2007 and opened up a practice in Lyon, France. This deep tissue massage technique is extremely efficient in correcting postural problems and enhancing physical performance. After 15 years in France, Peter moved back to Germany in 2016. He now runs a busy practice in Wiesbaden.

Peter now teaches Senmotic fighting techniques to private students and dedicates his time to his fascia therapy practice. He is also the official trainer for Senmotic fascia therapy in France and has trained a first generation of French practitioners.

In 2013 he published his acclaimed video course "Improve Your Posture Now (and Get Rid of Your Back Pain!), which has helped hundreds of people all over the world.

IMPROVE YOUR POSTURE AND GET RID OF YOUR BACK PAIN!

Life-changing stuff.

James Hollister

THE VIDEO COURSE ON POSTURE AND BACK PAIN

This course was created in 2013 and is the result of many years of working as fascia-therapist and teaching people how to have better posture. It brings all the concepts you learned in this book to life and allows for deeper understanding of the rules of good posture.

The course has since received outstanding ratings and incredible feedback from happy clients all over the world.

The course continues to grow in content and you can now discover the theory and practice of perfect posture on your own through these 45 simple exercises and explanations of basic anatomy and biomechanics. At the time of writing the course includes over three hours of video content.

The course comes complete with four additional e-books for more in-depth explanations.

The knowledge gained in this course will not only teach you how to live everyday life without pain, but how to thrive in activities or sports requiring balance and coordination. You will be able to run, dance, or practice martial arts once again - or just play with your children or grand-children.

Each section focuses on uniquely important aspects of your body.

1. You will learn how to breathe more easily and efficiently. Your breathing is the essence of your life. Take control of it and you will gain more energy.

2. You will learn how to stand for longer periods of time without pain. Control your pelvis and you control all of your movements. This exercise will improve your balance and stability. It will make you stronger and lower the danger of falling.

3. You will learn how to walk in a way that relaxes your spine and your lower back in particular. This knowledge is particularly useful in fighting lower back pain - you can be your own chiropractor.

4. You will learn how to sit straight without pain or effort. Sit actively to prevent back or shoulder injuries.

5. You will learn the ergonomics of the perfect working space. You will be able to work longer and stay more relaxed. Find the necessary energy to concentrate on your projects.

6. As you sleep six to nine hours every night, good sleeping posture is crucial in fixing your overall posture. Using a pillow under your head or choosing a bad mattress can cause serious health problems. This section will teach you how to correct and improve your posture during your sleep and how to choose the right mattress.

All these exercises and tips to fix your posture can also result in immediate pain relief. You can do these exercises in the comfort of your own home. They will take 5 to 15 minutes to do and you can expect to complete the program within about three weeks.

All of the exercises are easy and do not require any special skills for healthy individuals. The knowledge gained does not replace medical advice. In case of doubt, please consult your doctor.

If you are already working with a chiropractor or an osteopath, this program will complement your treatment.

As a Thank You for reading this book, you can find a discount page for the course on my website[10].

---

10   http://www.massage-therapy-wiesbaden.com

BAREFOOT SHOES – STRONG FEET FOR GOOD POSTURE

I bought my first pair of "healthy shoes" when I was 22 from a well-known German brand which makes flat shoes with enough room for the toes. They looked like my grandfather's shoes, only bigger. Thankfully, the sole broke after only six months. I learned only later that this brand has quality issues relating to their manufacture in India, but that aside, they were still far from perfect as the sole was way too thick. This was in the early nineties.

I forgot about healthy shoes for a while, but the question came back when I trained as a fascia therapist in 2007.

Even though new brands with thinner soles had hit the market, my colleagues and I still had trouble finding minimalistic shoes that would fit all our needs. One of the major problems was that most of these brands were pure plastic shoes, offering a very limited life expectancy and guaranteed smelly feet.

The issue of finding healthy shoes became even more urgent when I started working as a therapist and saw just how harmful "normal shoes" are to posture.

Fortunately, at that time, Frank Demann, founder of Senmotic blue fascia therapy and Senmotic red martial arts, decided to produce shoes that would not only meet our requirements as therapists, but also look like normal shoes that people older than sixteen could actually wear. Made in Germany, these shoes not only met our quality standards, but also guaranteed good working conditions and wages at a time when scandals concerning the manufacturing conditions for clothes and shoes in developing countries were starting to be reported in the media.

I remember the first time I wore them. I came home after a long walk, quite delighted with the barefoot experience and started going about my business.

It was only much later in the evening that I realized I had completely forgotten take my shoes off when I came in. This hadn't happened in years.

As you know from my chapter on shoes and walking, good shoes are a condition-sine-qua-non for having good posture in everyday life. They are in fact an essential investment.

Other good brands have hit the market since, but if you start looking into buying minimal shoe-wear, you can always start here: www.senmotic-shoes.eu.

SENMOTIC BLUE – FASCIA THERAPY

I had my first session of Senmotic blue fascia therapy in my early 30's. I didn't really know why I was there, since I was experiencing no particular pains or limitations and felt quite fit.

But my teacher, Frank Demann, had told me it would improve my martial arts skills and so I was happy to try it. Could you really change a person's posture or help him or her to move better with what I still thought was just a massage?

The first thing I noticed was that this had nothing to do with a massage, which is basically about working your muscles like bread dough.

Fascia therapy treats the connective tissue and feels completely different. It feels like your tissue melts under the hands, fists or elbows of the practitioner. Often much gentler, but sometimes much deeper and even slightly painful, you feel your tissue being stretched, almost ironed.

The first (of ten) sessions usually treats the torso and one of the expected benefits is that it gives your lungs more room to breathe.

My Eureka moment was when Frank worked on my diaphragm. His finger went under my ribs, caught hold of my diaphragm and gently pulled the tissue sideways.

For a second it felt like a side stitch, but then my rib cage heaved and breathed in as deeply as if I'd come up for air. It felt as if I had had a chain around my torso that had kept me from breathing for many years and I didn't even know it was there until the chain was taken off.

Connective tissue is like the fabric we make clothes from, in that its tightness can restrict movement. As your tissue becomes dry and sticks to other layers of tissue, your movement range decreases ever so slightly - but every day. The lucky one percent of older people who do not experience major restrictions of movement reminds us of the fact that this is not inevitable, but is to a large degree a question of exercise and, most of all, the quality of our every day movement.

Wear tight jeans or a shirt for any length of time and the tissue will restrict the amplitude of your movements. Senmotic blue feels like taking those clothes off and rediscovering how much room there is - inside yourself and out.

The connective tissue has many nerve endings, which allows the therapist to communicate directly with your nervous system. This way, the therapist not only works with your muscles and connective tissue, but also directly with your brain.

Many clients feel that this physical liberation also has emotional effects. While our work as therapists is purely mechanical, clients often tell us about life changes they have made during or after the ten-session cycle. They get out of toxic relationships, make important career changes or sometimes just stop worrying.

http://www.massage-therapy-wiesbaden.com for more information.